Believe it! Create a tailor-made treat-ment program by combining traditional cancer therapy with adjunct therapies—*practical procedures* that can help you or someone you love mobilize the immune system, stimulate the body—and *beat the odds!*

* DIET—How proper nutrition revives a weakened defense system
* EXERCISE THERAPY—Why chang-ing your metabolism can reverse the processes that create illness
* MEDITATION AND VISUALIZA-TION—Strengthening the mind–body link, the most powerful healing force at your disposal

PLUS

* HYPNOSIS
* NUTRITIONAL SUPPLEMENTS
* HOW TO SYSTEMATICALLY COM-BINE THESE METHODS WITH TRA-DITIONAL MEDICAL CARE
* TRUE, INSPIRATIONAL ACCOUNTS OF PATIENTS' SUCCESSES
* COMPLETE BIBLIOGRAPHY AND SOURCE LISTINGS

"Provocative!"—*Booklist*

BEATING The ODDS

ALTERNATIVE TREATMENTS THAT HAVE WORKED MIRACLES AGAINST CANCER

ALBERT MARCHETTI, M.D.

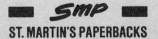

ST. MARTIN'S PAPERBACKS

This book is about cancer and the mysterious cures known as spontaneous remissions. But more than this, it is about power. The tremendous power of lightning and thunder. The power of an ocean wave crashing on the shore. The power of a million suns blazing in the sky. The amazing power of the human mind and body to regenerate. The power of nature. The power of understanding, compassion, and love.

The information contained in this book is for educational purposes only. Anyone wishing to use it in a practical manner should do so only with the guidance and supervision of a trained professional. Information on specific treatment centers, clinics, and practitioners is provided to give the reader a wide range of therapeutic choices, but these names should not be considered recommendations.

Published by arrangement with Contemporary Books

BEATING THE ODDS

Copyright © 1988 by Albert Marchetti, M.D.

Library of Congress Catalog Card Number: 88-7069

ISBN: 0-312-92236-1

Printed in the United States of America

St. Martin's Press hardcover edition published 1988
St. Martin's Paperbacks edition/July 1990

10 9 8 7 6 5 4 3 2 1

Preface

From the conception of this book in 1984, I have been privileged to work with a great number of people who have decided to help along their cures. My patients' successes have ranged from continued combat to complete cure and more than twenty years of remission. Some of the people with whom I became involved particularly touched me, not only because of the pain of their struggles, but also because of their perseverance and determination to survive. For some of these people, the road to remission was smooth; for others it was and still is rocky. But each has managed to beat the odds.

In a recent case, one of extreme circumstances, the patient came to me after his personal physician found an inordinately aggressive tumor, a mixed sarcoma, attached to vital organs in the patient's abdomen. When the tumor was first discovered, it was already the size of a grapefruit, and it was growing rapidly. A search of the finest doctor to handle the case led us to a large metropolitan cancer center, where several hours of complicated surgery were required to remove the large mass. Although the surgery seemed successful, the pathology report was unkind. Some of the tumor had been left behind. Doctors began radiation and chemotherapy, and I worked with the patient on a combined program of dietary modification and exercise. The patient followed the adjunct program for two years and seemed to progress well. The patient went through a period of complacency, and then a setback occurred. Cancer developed elsewhere in his body. More chemotherapy was ordered, and the patient rededicated himself to the adjunct program, which was, of course, modified to counterbalance the unfortunate turn of events. I added visualization to high doses of vitamin C to better the therapeutic results of the chemotherapy and to ease its side effects. Now, with the completion of another year, the tumor is beginning to shrink. The celebration of a recent birthday (66) marked the fourth year of survival for a patient who carried a prognosis of only a few months.

Another patient I have had the pleasure of working with lives in Tampa, Florida. Six months ago I had the difficult task of informing him that his blood tests indicated the possibility of blood cancer and required further evaluation. A subsequent marrow biopsy revealed a leukemia, but I told him he shouldn't worry because I thought there was a good chance the cancer could be controlled without even conventional therapy (something I certainly do not recommend in all cases). With the applied therapies of vitamin supplementation, dietary modification, and enhanced physical activity, he has managed to restrain the progress of his illness. Continued testing has revealed a gradual but continual reduction of his white blood cell count to almost normal levels.

Finally, this past Thanksgiving I spoke again with a remarkable patient for whom I had consulted over the years. More than fifteen years ago, she underwent surgery for a cancer of the intestinal tract. As with my patient with the aggressive tumor, the pathology department reported that some of the cancer had been left behind. In this particular case, in accordance with the family's wishes, the patient was not informed of this complication, but was led to believe that the operation had been a complete success. Still, wishing to eliminate the conditions that had originally brought about her illness, the woman underwent a complete revision of her diet to eliminate fats, sweets, meat, and other foods that are today considered unhealthy. In addition, she began to participate in a program of daily exercise that included social sports. When she contacted me, her perseverance had already paid off. Today, she is a vigorous, youthful woman, still adhering to the combined prescription of diet and exercise I've recommended and, remarkably, never spending another minute treating the complications of the residual cancer. She's been in remission for years!

The efforts of the patient truly count and, perhaps more than any other factor in the treatment of cancer, determine the ultimate outcome of therapy. It is to these people and others like them who have managed to beat the odds through their own persistence and will to survive that I dedicate this book.

Contents

Acknowledgments

Sincere appreciation to all those whose faith and support brought this work to fruition:

- John Cushing, who gave friendship, encouragement, and creative inspiration

- Barney Zinger, who offered interest, comments, and motivation

- Kenneth Moses, who lent his support, spirituality, and sense of humanity

- Francis Marincola, who provided tenacity and moral support

- Peter Miller, who expended great energy and effort in my behalf

And a very special thanks to Stacy Prince, my wonderful editor at Contemporary Books, whose belief in the project not only made it happen, but also made it shine. I am forever indebted to her for the inspiration and direction she gave and the incredible patience she demonstrated.

Introduction

In the medical profession, the words *remission* or *spontaneous remission* signify the automatic and complete recovery from cancer, a sometimes unexpected and mysterious event. They are the words most joyfully spoken by cancer specialists and most graciously received by cancer patients. They are the words that indicate a complete cure, a triumph over illness. They are the words that give new life. Within the pages of this book, you will explore numerous real-life examples of "spontaneous remissions" and discover the ultimate cause behind each of them. You will see how ordinary people managed to change the course of their illnesses by altering their mental attitude and physical makeup. Finally, you will learn about the actual techniques and methods that have been shown to bring about complete and lasting cures—practical procedures that can shift the odds of recovery in your favor and make the difference between life and death.

While this book is specifically addressed to the individual who carries the diagnosis of cancer and who is searching for a successful and lasting cure, it can be equally valuable to the patient's family and friends who want to help in any way possible but lack the knowledge to do so. Additionally, it will serve health-conscious people who desire to educate themselves and initiate or perfect a sound approach to cancer prevention and health maintenance.

The information and case studies presented within these pages are well supported by four years of exhaustive research and an ongoing review of the world literature. From the concept of spontaneous remission to the discussions on DNA, interferon, natural killer cells, and natural cancer defense, each topic will carry you further down the road of understanding. At the end of that road, you will have the knowledge and information you need to wisely select therapies most suitable for you.

The therapies described in this book are intended as adjuncts to, not substitutes for, the three most common cancer treatments: surgery, chemotherapy, and radiation. What you will discover here are a host of other catalysts that propel patients into remission, therapies like visualization, macrobiotics, meditation, and exercise. They are all presented so that you can tailor a specific, powerful program from the widest possible selection of alternatives and use it in conjunction with expert medical care.

Just as important, the information presented in this book is inspirational. Each chapter provides not only knowledge but also hope. Each case history illustrates that we all naturally possess the substances, cells, and elements needed to bring on a remission. As you read about the many adjunct therapies and the precise methods that generate remission, you will be exhilarated and motivated to act.

Consider the benefits of each adjunct therapy and appraise your own ability and desire to learn the techniques and persevere in the program. At the same time, attempt to evaluate your life in terms of philosophy and spirituality, stress and anxiety, nutrition and activity. This will help you to select the therapies that best address your specific needs and abilities. Once you have made your selections, be sure to obtain professional help and learn as much as possible about the specific self-treatments you have chosen. With all the energy you can summon, you must then perform the techniques and practices to the best of your ability, day in and day out, until you obtain the results you desire.

While this task may seem formidable, it is not without immediate gratification. From the very beginning of a well-formulated adjunct program, you will start to feel better, emotionally and physically. With each passing day, you will gain control over life events and the course the disease will take. As you develop a new inner strength, the effects of the program will become more obvious, constantly generating more and more positive results until you achieve the ultimate goal of remission. The entire process becomes a controllable event, dependent only on your ability to push the right buttons by choosing the appropriate therapies and applying them with total conviction and dedication. The commitment must be life-long, but its reward is life itself.

So read with care and attention, reflect on your condition and its probable causes, and then choose your therapies well. By helping yourself and applying the principles presented in this book, you will greatly increase your odds of achieving a remission and a total cancer cure.

1
The Spontaneous Remission of Cancer

REMISSION OF LIVER CANCER IN A FIVE-MONTH-OLD INFANT

Twenty-five years after liver cancer was diagnosed in an infant boy, the patient seemed to have beaten the odds against his survival and was reported to be "in good health and gainfully employed." His case had been reviewed in a follow-up study by three physicians: William J. McSweeny, Kevin E. Bove, and James Mac-Adams from the departments of radiology, pathology, and pediatrics at the University of Cincinnati College of Medicine. The findings were unusual.

At the time of the original diagnosis, the patient was just five and a half months old. He was brought to the Cincinnati Children's Hospital in June 1946 with a large abdominal mass and severe anemia. His tumor was so large that it literally filled the entire right side of his abdomen, extending from the ribs to the pelvis. His stomach and intestines were completely displaced to the left, pressing against the rib cage.

Because of the severity of his condition, the child was immediately scheduled for exploratory surgery to de-

5

termine the nature and extent of the problem. In the operating room, a generous abdominal incision revealed a dark red tumor that appeared to completely occupy the liver. A biopsy was taken, and the incision was closed. The tumor was too large to remove.

After recovering from the surgery, the infant was sent home with a hopeless diagnosis. Tissue studies of the biopsy indicated hepatoma—cancer of the liver—and since no therapy was given, the child was expected to die. But sometimes a patient's outcome is unexpected. Surprisingly, the child improved.

Two years after surgery, the child was reexamined, and the liver was greatly diminished. X-rays still demonstrated a large liver mass, but it was certainly smaller than before. Much of it was replaced with calcium deposits.

At age eight, another series of x-rays was taken, and the tumor was even smaller. There were more areas of calcification, and the tumor had become denser as it shrank.

At age twenty-five, when the patient was last seen, he was reported to be "in good health and gainfully employed." The physical examination turned up no unusual findings, and the liver, although slightly nodular and contracted, showed no evidence of the tumor.

Although the doctors who reviewed the case in 1971 agreed that the patient did indeed have a tumor in the liver when he was an infant, they contested the 1946 diagnosis of hepatoma-type liver cancer. Instead, they favored "hemangioendothelioma," a blood-vessel tumor that had grown within the liver.

These diagnoses are significantly different. With hepatomas, children usually die. With hemangioendotheliomas, they generally live. Regardless, the tumor had not been treated because the case was considered hopeless at the time. Yet twenty-five years later, the five-month-old baby boy who had been discharged from the hospital as a terminal cancer patient was a grown man, tumor-free, in good health, and gainfully employed. Without any therapy, he was cured of a tumor that had completely filled his abdomen and threatened his very existence. Without any treatment, a massive tumor had calcified, shrunk, and just disappeared. Amazing!

REMISSION OF CANCER FOLLOWING MEASLES INFECTION

In another case, the patient was an eight-year-old African boy who entered Mulago Hospital (Uganda) on December 1, 1970, with a form of cancer known as Burkett's lymphoma—a malignant condition of the lymph glands. The case was reported in the July 10, 1971, issue of *The Lancet*, a highly respected British medical journal, and the research was supported by the National Cancer Institute in Bethesda, Maryland.

At the time of the boy's admission, the malignancy was growing behind his right eye, causing blindness, paralysis, and displacement of the eye. A biopsy of the tumor was performed, and when the abnormal tissue was prepared and examined under a microscope, it was described as Burkett's lymphoma, a horrible form of cancer.

To complicate matters, on December 13, before any kind of therapy could be initiated, the child caught the measles. Also on that day, his doctors noted that the tumor behind his eye had begun to shrink. After just two weeks, the measles infection cleared—and the tumor had totally disappeared. Completely and without any form of therapy, the child was cured.

Apparently there was a connection between the infection and the disappearance of the tumor. But what was the connection? Did the measles virus attack the tumor cells? Did the body's reaction to the measles provoke a reaction to the tumor? What caused the cure? Was it fever, antibodies, interferon, or steroids produced and released from the adrenal glands?

Avrum Z. Bluming and John L. Zeigler, who reported

this case from the Uganda Cancer Institute at Kampala, Uganda, were uncertain about the relationship between the measles and the tumor, but they were convinced that the child was totally free of cancer.

REMISSION OF STOMACH CANCER THAT HAD SPREAD TO THE LIVER

At the age of fifty-one, a patient was admitted to Peter Bent Brigham Hospital in Boston. He had been drinking heavily—three to four fifths of whiskey each week—and was troubled by stomach problems, weight loss, and fatigue. The doctors launched a full investigation, and when the patient finally went to exploratory surgery, they discovered and removed a stomach tumor they described as "fist size." In addition, they removed enlarged lymph glands around the stomach and biopsied abnormal nodules in the liver. The pathology department confirmed the diagnosis. The tumor was an adenocarcinoma of the stomach, or simply stomach cancer. And although the lymph glands contained no cancer, a microscopic study of the liver biopsy was positive for adenocarcinoma, just like the cancer removed from the stomach. The cancer had already spread and occupied the liver.

In 1956, when this case occurred, removing the cancer from the stomach was considered difficult, although surgically possible. However, removing the cancer from the liver was impossible because today's techniques of radio- and chemotherapy were then virtually unknown. Therefore, at the time of the diagnosis, the prognosis was grave, and the case was considered terminal.

Then, unexpectedly, on the tenth day after surgery, the patient developed an infection within his abdomen and underwent a second operation to drain an abscess that developed around the stomach incision where the cancer had been cut away. The good news: the infection quickly cleared, and the patient left the hospital. The bad news: although both surgeries were successful, the patient was still doomed to die because he still had cancer in his liver.

But the patient didn't die!

Five months after his discharge from the hospital, he had gained twenty pounds and had returned to work symptom-free, a hopeful sign. Three years later, however, he developed a small mass in his neck and returned to the hospital for an evaluation. Although his doctors believed that the mass represented a further manifestation of the cancer, they did nothing. The case was already considered terminal because of the liver metastases, so, they reasoned, why put the patient through unnecessary discomfort in his last days?

Then circumstances began to change. Two years after the neck mass developed, it mysteriously and spontaneously disappeared. By 1968, twelve years after the double surgeries, the patient seemed totally cured. While the patient was undergoing unrelated gallbladder surgery for gallstones, the surgeons completely reexamined him inside and out and found him to be totally free of cancer. No nodules in the liver. No recurrent cancer in the stomach. No cancer in the neck. In fact, the doctors found no cancer whatsoever.

After reviewing the case and examining all the reports, slides, lab work, and x-rays, Steven A. Rosenberg, Edward Fox, and Winthroup H. Churchill of the National Cancer Institute in Bethesda, Maryland, submitted their report to *Cancer* magazine, where it was published in February 1972. The doctors concluded, "The patient provides evidence that the regression of hepatic metastases from stomach cancer can occur without therapy." They added, "The cause of such regression is unknown." Regardless, the patient was fully recovered and cancer-free.

REMISSION OF METASTATIC CANCER OF THE TESTICLE

Another story involves a thirty-four-year-old man whose enlarged left testicle was caused by a tumor. During surgery, his doctors removed his cancer by removing his testicle. In addition, to make sure all of the cancer was excised or destroyed, the patient received radiation therapy before returning home. All seemed well.

However, six months after his optimistic release from the hospital, he had a serious reversal. Back pain forced a return to the hospital and a reevaluation. This time, his doctors discovered tumor nodules in his lungs. They decided that the lung tumors were most likely distant extensions of the original testicular cancer, either not present or too small to be noticed in previous x-rays. Regardless, the medical odds certainly favored the doctors' diagnosis of "multiple lung metastases" of the primary tumor of the testes. So the once hopeful patient suddenly had a hopeless future, especially since the original radiation therapy had failed to kill the cancer cells that now grew abundantly in his lungs.

No therapy was given because, in the opinion of his doctors, no therapy would work. Surgery was out of the question; there were too many nodules in too many places. And how many more would develop? Radiation therapy had already proved ineffective. Other forms of therapy remained undiscovered back in 1963, when this case was documented at the Christie Hospital and Holt Radium Institute of Manchester, England. So the patient was released from the institute with the news that he was going to die because there was no appropriate treatment for him.

But the patient didn't die. He continued to live for two more years and was completely reexamined for the third time in August 1965. At that time, his chest x-rays were much improved; the lung nodules were smaller, and some had actually disappeared.

Six more months passed, and he was still alive. New x-rays showed even further reduction in the size and number of lung nodules. Finally, by December 1975 he was totally cured. Although he had never been treated for metastatic tumors in his lungs, complete reexaminations proved beyond the shadow of a doubt that he was free of cancer.

The cases just discussed are but four isolated examples of what is known as spontaneous remission: the total and sometimes inexplicable cure of cancer. Nothing is unique about these cases, but they are all special in that they illustrate an important point: *Spontaneous remissions really occur. Cancer can be healed naturally.*

If just one case were presented here, if only one spontaneous cancer cure had been discovered and then documented, that would be enough to give hope. But the fact is, thousands of spontaneous cures have been reported throughout the world. And more are occurring all the time.

As early as the turn of the century, scientists and doctors recognized and described the phenomenon of spontaneous remission. In 1903, the "spontaneous healing of cancer" was noted in Germany. In 1906, the "spontaneous cure of cancer" was recorded in the United States. A "natural cancer cure" was highlighted in 1912 in the British medical literature. In 1921, doctors wrote, "Not only may the metastases be held in check, but they may actually recede and disappear." By 1950 they went so far as to note, "Malignant neoplasms undergo periods of spontaneous arrest and regression."

Before a 1956 meeting of the Canadian Association of Radiologists, William Boyd, a noted medical doctor and eloquent lecturer and teacher, dramatically stated:

We know that while some cancers are fearfully rapid in their course, others are incredibly slow. A slow-growing tumor may suddenly start to grow faster, while, on the other hand, the growth of a tumor may [actually] slow down. Finally, growth may stop completely and the cancer may resolve and eventually disappear. To shut our eyes and refuse to believe in spontaneous regression and recovery from cancer is absurd.

While the observations and comments of Dr. Boyd and his predecessors were factual and far-reaching, they were also a bit premature. Many cases had been reported since the turn of the century, but when Dr. Boyd presented his illuminating lecture in 1956, few reports had been fully researched and accurately documented. In many cases, existing diagnostic techniques were inadequate to identify the illness accurately, or thorough investigations were never performed, leaving the researcher to ponder the possibility of misdiagnosis and misinterpretation. These problems delayed widespread interest and acceptance for another decade.

Then in the mid-1960s a truly exhaustive study was undertaken. Two American doctors, Tilden C. Everson and Warren H. Cole, collected and reviewed the world literature on the subject and compiled a wealth of data, which they formally presented to the international medical community in 1966. Entitled *Spontaneous Regression of Cancer*, their milestone book provided undeniable evidence of the reality of spontaneous cancer cures. Here's why:

Of the hundreds, perhaps thousands, of cases they reviewed, only indisputable examples were accepted. The cases were considered only if tissue studies had been performed, absolutely verifying the diagnosis of cancer.

Likewise, only reports of cancers that disappeared on their own were included—that is, cases that had received absolutely no treatment or what is today considered inadequate treatment. Consequently, the only possible cause for cure in each case was the natural healing power of the body itself. Recovery was truly unaided and spontaneous.

People of all ages, males, females, blacks, whites, Asians, Americans, Africans, and Europeans were included. All types of cancers were discussed and were shown to resolve on their own. Kidney cancer, neuroblastoma, malignant melanoma, choriocarcinoma, bladder cancer, soft-tissue sarcoma, bone cancer, rectal cancer, breast cancer—the list seemed endless.

Now the words of Dr. Boyd had renewed meaning. "To shut our eyes and refuse to believe in spontaneous regression and recovery from cancer is absurd." Spontaneous remissions are an established medical fact, as real and tangible as the book you hold in your hands.

Armed with this knowledge, you are ready to battle your own illness or protect yourself from the threat of disease, knowing full well that you already possess the necessary weapons to maintain good health. Spontaneous remissions are not miracles; they are the natural consequence of a cause-and-effect process, an interplay between you and your health. Spontaneous remissions are an indication that the human body, by combining its own natural defense system with a person's will and desire, can triumph over illness. You already have the mechanisms to cure yourself of any disease, including cancer. Now it's up to you to bring these natural agents into play.

"But am I capable of doing this?" you might ask. And if so, "Will I be able to experience a remission?"

The answer to these questions is an emphatic *yes*. In fact, you have already experienced the phenomenon many times. You simply have not been aware of it. It may seem incredible, but we all undergo spontaneous remissions, constantly, perhaps every single day of our lives, as our natural defense system fights a never-ending battle against cancer and disease.

Our bodies are in a perpetual state of change. Old cells die and are replaced by new cells at a rate of billions per day. Injuries are repaired. New tissues form. Growth transpires. These are everyday occurrences needed to rejuvenate our bodies. But the process doesn't work perfectly every time. Cell repair is occasionally incomplete or imprecise, new tissues may form erratically, and cell reproduction is periodically altered. When these things happen, they can cause problems. One of those problems is cancer.

Most cancers begin as a single cell or group of cells that develops in an unusual manner. Cell reproductive and growth processes mutate and start to function in a bizarre way, creating new cells that are abnormal and lead to tumors. Our natural defense systems have to immediately identify and eliminate these abnormal cells. In daily battles, we regularly meet the challenge and overcome the deadly malignant foe, experiencing routine spontaneous remissions in the process. *From our earliest days of childhood through our adult lives, this process is repeated over and over again.* It's inherent in our physical makeup; it is part of our normal functions. It's as natural as eating, breathing, and sleeping.

As you progress through this book and gain a better understanding of the malignant process and the reactions of the natural defense system to cancer and all other diseases, you will come to appreciate the great power that is in your command and you will discover how to use that power to your good. You will learn about methods that have worked for other people, methods that have brought the natural defense system to a point of excellence in restoring and maintaining good health. From real examples, you will learn to greatly increase your odds of survival or longevity by doing only those things that truly come naturally.

I
HOW HEALING
WORKS

2
The Process of Healing

In a desperate yet faithful search for a life-saving cure, Vittorio Micheli, a soldier in the Italian army, traveled to the Roman Catholic shrine of Lourdes in southern France. Thirteen months previously, he had been informed that a malignant tumor, a sarcoma, was growing in his left pelvis. As the tumor continued to enlarge with each passing day, Micheli grew more and more troubled about his fate. His general health was rapidly deteriorating, he had lost a lot of weight, and the expanding tumor was gradually separating his leg from his hip joint. Upon his arrival at the holy shrine, he could not walk, stand, or even control his leg, which for support had to be bound in a full-length cast. His condition was, in fact, so grave that he needed physical assistance to lower himself into the curative waters of the healing shrine.

But his life was about to change.

After only a few immersions in the holy waters, Micheli noted a metamorphosis. First of all, his appetite returned to normal after many months of anorexia and physical wasting. This in itself may have been a life-saving change, since his body desperately needed nourishment. Second, the pain in his hip, which had been steadily increasing over the course of the illness, suddenly and without explanation, disappeared. Without any medication whatsoever, the young Italian soldier was pain-free. Then Micheli perceived the bones of his hip, pelvis, and femur to be actually reuniting, growing back together to form a new hip joint.

Upon Micheli's return home, he immediately reported the good news to his doctors. They expressed complete skepticism in the cure, believing that a sarcoma of the pelvis could not resolve without any therapy and in such a short time. Contradicting Micheli's beliefs, they insisted that he retain his cast in order to keep his leg and pelvis attached. They unanimously concurred that his death was imminent, an expected consequence of a deadly disease. But the hopeful Micheli continued not only to live but also to improve. Within the short period of one month, he was walking around on his own. Suffice it to say, his doctors were amazed.

In an attempt to explain the unlikely chain of events, the skeptical physicians ordered an x-ray. It clearly showed that where a large fulminating tumor mass had been, there was only the residue of a burned-out cancer. Where the hip had been pushed apart by the cancerous growth, there was renewed bone growth and the possibility of a complete reunion. Indeed, the tumor had truly shrunk, and the bones were actually reuniting. To the great joy of young Micheli, recovery continued over the next five years, and continuous medical follow-up over the same period confirmed that the tumor had completely disappeared and the pelvis had fully returned to normal. Without any medical therapy, Vittorio Micheli, a youthful soldier who placed his faith in the hands of the Lord, was totally free of cancer and restored to his natural state of good health.

Although this case is impressive by virtue of its dramatic reversal of events and conditions, it is but one twentieth-century cure from the healing shrine of Lourdes. There are many others, and there is also real documentation of the healing power. Years ago, to confirm the legitimacy of recoveries, a medical committee was established at the holy shrine for the purpose of examining and documenting all cures. The members of the International Medical Association of Lourdes meticulously record each occurrence, and their investigations are open for review. Cases like Micheli's are rare, but they have been recorded. Thanks to the power of the healing waters and the grace of God, miracles do occur, and lives are spared.

But are they really miracles, these unusual cures, these magical metamorphoses that transform individuals and turn sickness into health and near death into new life?

While natural cancer cures are seen as odd occurrences, even miracles, most other examples of the body's ability to heal itself are taken for granted. For example, is it so remarkable that a cut heals or an infection clears? Is it really incredible that measles and chicken pox run their course, only to be ultimately conquered by a competent immune system? What's so miraculous about a bone that breaks and then mends? If these are all natural occurrences, examples of the body's ability to heal itself, then what's so special about the body's ability to dissipate cancer? The true miracle is the innate power of our bodies, not only to repair but actually to regenerate, not only to heal but genuinely to return to normal. That's the true miracle, and it's really no miracle at all, other than the miracle of life itself.

Considering Vittorio Micheli's case and the other examples of remissions cited earlier, it is obvious that the body truly has the ability to heal itself of cancer. When a five-month-old child dissolves a liver tumor or a fifty-one-year-old man rids his body of widely disseminated stomach cancer, both without the aid of adequate medical treatment, the body's natural self-healing power is at work. New examples arise daily as people from all walks of life profess to being cured through some form of self-directed therapy.

Scientists believe that, in all cases of unexplained recoveries, normal healing processes are the cause. Never has there been a scientifically documented case of some otherworldly cause for an outstanding cure. If anything special occurred in any exceptional case, it was the rate of cure, not the means.

According to Alexis Carrel, who has observed and reported on the Lourdes "miracles," there is really nothing special about the great majority of them. They would have happened anyway, as the natural resolutions of common diseases. In a very small number of cases like Micheli's, where healing was unusual or extraordinary in some way, Carrel explained that although the process was natural, the rate of cure was somehow greatly accelerated.

Ailon Shiloh of the University of South Florida tends to agree with Carrel's observations. Shiloh, a recognized expert on faith healing, has witnessed innumerable cases in which illnesses and cures were both real. According to his observations, several ingredients are necessary to a successful faith healing. They include:

- A condition that is reversible. For example, an amputated leg never regrows, and an enucleated eye never regenerates. Only amenable illnesses have the potential to be cured.

- The healer must be a forgiving parental figure whose love, faith, and absolution inspire the ill to make a change.

- The event must be witnessed by a host of spiritual supporters whose active encouragement creates the necessary excitement and fervor.

• The surroundings or the occasion must have a special significance, as do the Holy Shrine of Lourdes and the annual sunrise ceremony of a healing ministry.

• Most importantly, the devotees must have supreme faith in the power of the healer and the entire healing process, plus an overwhelming desire to be cured. They fully place themselves in God's hands and allow the Lord to act for them. When these conditions exist and the person to be cured achieves an unusual state of spirituality, the healing takes place. It is natural healing, using the normal processes of the body, but it is much accelerated and highly concentrated and specific, stimulated by the powerful belief that God has intervened and has directed the cure.

In cases of total remission from cancer, the cause of the cure is completely natural, regardless of the forces that inspire or direct the event. Most likely, the immune system peaks in performance, sparked by some special sequence of events. The chemicals of well-being are released in abundance. White blood cells surge to fight the malignant foe. Antibodies are produced. Interferon floods the body. The tumor is destroyed. This is the natural chain of events. This is natural healing—only it occurs with blazing speed.

With these important thoughts in mind, a critical question arises, a question that directs the course of medical investigation and treatment in this country and around the world. It pertains to every one of us and can literally mean the difference between life and death for millions of people, now and to come: Can the entire healing process, our natural ability to rid the body of disease, be mentally controlled, directed by will? Can we consciously control our own natural defense systems and focus the life-saving forces that exist within us? It may seem incredible, but for the first time in modern medical history, doctors are beginning to agree that, yes, we can.

With the most sophisticated tools and techniques ever known, researchers continue to open new areas of understanding the healing cells and substances present within us. From the pages of the latest research papers and the journals of experimental medicine come ever increasing reports of the power of the human mind and body to reverse disease. People of all races and nationalities have testified to cures of their physical problems through self-generated healing. All evidence points to one inescapable conclusion: We can make deliberate adjustments in our lives and direct the life forces of our bodies.

To accomplish these lifesaving tasks yourself, you must first be critically aware of the circumstances in your life that brought about your illness. You must understand the physical and emotional causes of cancer so that you will know what aspects of your life need changing. You must comprehend the processes by which cancer is naturally controlled within your body. This information is provided for you on the pages of this book. As you read each chapter, reflect on your own condition. By connecting the ideas here with your experiences, you should be able to select the self-initiated therapies that will slow, stop, or even reverse the course of your disease.

This is, indeed, wonderful news. Yet it requires your active participation. To free yourself from the bondage of your illness, you must make a valiant and dedicated effort to achieve your own cure. You must embark on an awesome journey that brings you into contact with your innermost feelings and with the external forces that play upon your life. In a spirit of true heroism and with the desire to meet and conquer not only your illness but also your fears and doubts, you must face yourself and say: I have the power to do all things and be all things, and nothing will stand in my way.

This is the winning attitude. It is the common denominator in most of the exceptional patients who beat the odds and triumph over their illnesses. For some people it comes naturally, for others, it must be learned. This attitude can be subtle and silent or bold and boisterous, but regardless, it is probably the most important single requirement in directing a cure. This overwhelming desire to win the battle against your disease is a necessary ingredient of your success. Assume this attitude immediately. Carry it with you always, and let it fill your mind and body with an unshakable feeling of confidence.

Equally important is an absolute faith in your ability to achieve your goal of complete remission. You must truly and fully believe that you can beat the odds, that you have the inherent means of reversing your illness, and that you will be the deciding factor in your cure. Like the faith of the sick and worn Italian soldier in the healing waters of the holy shrine of Lourdes, your faith will make your efforts count. It will be the driving force behind the therapies that you choose. It will inspire you to go further and to achieve more. It will be the voice inside your head that says you can do it.

As you will see in the upcoming chapters, you already possess the means to cure yourself of cancer and most other illnesses. Before leaving the womb, you started to develop the elements of a natural defense system that is fine-tuned to identify, attack, and destroy malignant invaders in the body. These are God-given tools, sharpened through millions of years of evolution to be more effective than a surgeon's blade in removing cancerous growths forever. Now you must learn to bring these forces into play.

To effect a cure, you should do several important things. The first is to get the best medical or surgical assistance you can find. Probably you're already under the treatment of a doctor. If you suspect you have cancer and are not under the care of a doctor, seeing a physician must be your first step. The next chapter will give you some guidelines and resources for ensuring that you receive the best traditional care possible.

Second, you must develop a clear understanding of what cancer is and is not, and why your actions can make a difference. Chapters 4, 5, and 6 will help prove to you the amazing ability of your body to cure itself and the power of your mind to effect that cure. These chapters will aid you in developing a strong belief in your amazing potential for healing.

Third, you should read about the many adjunct therapies discussed in Chapters 7 through 13 and see which appeal to you. You may find more than one appealing.

Fourth, choose a therapy or combination of therapies and find one or more professionals in these areas who can help tailor a program especially for you. Although I have provided ample information on each adjunct therapy to give you an idea of how it works and how to do it, the best way to educate yourself is to read as much material as you can get your hands on, then to apply the knowledge you gain to create a program ideally suited to your personality and physiology. In Chapter 14, you will find suggestions for making sure that your traditional doctor and your adjunct therapists work together to get you better.

Last, and perhaps most important, comes your dedication. As you read the case histories in this book, you'll realize that almost every person who succeeds in curing his or her cancer is dedicated to the fight. These people follow their plans to the letter, and if their condition gets worse, they only try harder.

You can do it, too.

3
Conventional Therapy

A SUPER START

The diagnosis of cancer carries with it numerous critical decisions that must be made quickly and surely. The ultimate outcome of therapy often rests on these vital decisions. The reasons for choosing the finest medical and surgical care are obvious. Poor choices in the beginning lead to poor results in the end. Too many patients have said they only wished they had checked out their options further and made better choices at the start. So take time to learn about your problem, communicate often and in depth with your primary physician, and investigate your options thoroughly before you make your final decisions.

The first question you must ask your doctor is how much time you have to make the necessary treatment decisions. Based on the nature of the malignancy, the doctor will know the usual course of the disease and can provide you with a reasonable timetable. For example, if you have carcinoma in situ of the cervix, you have ample time to select the right approach to treatment.

However, if you have a choriocarcinoma of the testis, you must be more aggressive in making immediate arrangements for therapy, because even a slight delay could make a big difference.

Before you do anything, though, you must be certain of the diagnosis, and it is wise to get a second opinion right away. Do this at an established cancer treatment center or major hospital or university medical center. If you live in an area without such a facility, you must seek out the closest available location that has a reputation for diagnosing and treating cancer.

From your doctor and from the cancer center, request the following information:

- A specific diagnosis, including type and stage of the cancer

- The primary site of the tumor—exactly where it is located, in which organ or area of the body

- Where the cancer has spread. Is it confined to the primary location, or has it extended to other areas of the body?

- How fast it appears to be growing. What is the natural growth rate of similar tumors?

- A list of all the examinations, tests, and procedures that have been performed and the results of each

Be prepared for a minor battle in obtaining all of your reports. Many doctors are reluctant to release documents and data to their patients and occasionally decline requests. Others unselfishly share information and will cooperate to the fullest. Regardless, you must have free access to the results of all your tests in order to proceed efficiently in your quest for proper treatment and cure. If a problem arises, calmly explain to the reluctant physician that you appreciate his or her efforts in your behalf but simply need your results for further consultations. Ultimately, everyone will cooperate.

SELECTING A PHYSICIAN

Once you have obtained this information, you will be able to intelligently present yourself and your problem to the physician who will treat you. Your next objective is therefore to find the doctor most qualified to treat your problem. Generally, your quest will take you back to a large community hospital, university medical complex, comprehensive cancer treatment center, or perhaps a proficient private practitioner who comes well recommended. Although the task to find the best is laborious and exacting, some helpful sources of information are available:

- *Cancer Information Service.* Maintained by the National Cancer Institute, the Cancer Information Service is a toll-free line that provides patients with information about diagnosis and treatment, rehabilitation, and counseling. Call 800 information for the correct number for your area.

- *The American Cancer Society.* The American Cancer Society has chapters in most major U.S. cities and headquarters in New York City. Services provided include information about most cancers and therapies. Recently, the society published a book on diagnosis and treatment of all cancers. It is an excellent means of self-education, although slightly difficult for nonmedical personnel to comprehend. Local chapters of the society can direct patients to competent physicians and treatment centers and aid in transportation, home health care, and many other services.

- *Directories. The American Medical Directory* is a national directory of doctors and specialists. It is useful in identifying the doctors in your area who specialize in your type of problem. Listed are their names and credentials, along with their experience and medical credits. You can find this directory, along with a similar book, the *Directory of Medical Specialists*, at your local library. Look for surgeons, radiologists, and oncologists, depending on your specific needs. Later, this chapter describes the role of each of these specialists.

Although these directories contain a mass of information, they really don't indicate the "best" doctors and are difficult to use as a source of physician referrals. However, they can be used to evaluate the doctors that have been recommended to you, and you can feel secure that the doctors who are listed are well qualified to perform their specialties. With time and work, you can make specific selections from these books and further research the physicians whose names you have isolated. If they are inappropriate, they certainly should be able to provide excellent referrals to appropriate doctors.

Once you have located the names of several doctors who are capable of treating you, you should examine their personal histories. To check out a physician's reputation, you can call the hospital's department head in that specialty, the hospital administrator, or the head of the hospital review board. Sometimes these people will provide information. More often, people who work closely with your potential physician can give you insight into his or her abilities. Nurses and assistants, more than any others, have seen the doctor perform and know the quality of his or her work. They will usually speak frankly and honestly. Simply call the hospital, explain your situation, and ask for advice. The nurse, intern, resident, or assistant should be able to help.

Your primary physician frequently recommends other doctors to consult and treat you. This is certainly accepted practice, especially if your primary doctor is an expert in the field. After all, your doctor wants to achieve success in your case (that's to his or her credit) and will want to be assisted by the finest doctors available. Still, if you exercise due diligence in investigating all the doctors who are recommended, you will boost your confidence in the final outcome of treatment and help assure excellent results.

Surgeons

The primary treatment for most cancers is surgery, therefore, most patients will have to find a surgeon for treatment. The best doctor will have board certification in the particular field that encompasses your problem, and his or her reputation will be impeccable. For example, if the problem is cancer of the colon, you should seek out a gastroenterologist who is board certified in that field and has a fine surgical reputation. Better yet, the doctor should have advanced training in oncology (cancer therapy) and board certification in that field too. This dual certification means the doctor has trained and passed examinations in gastroenterology and oncology.

Radiologists

There are two general fields of radiology: diagnostic radiology and therapeutic radiology. The first uses x-ray techniques to diagnose disease; the second actually treats disease with radiation. If you are advised to complete a course of radiotherapy, it is the second type of radiologist with whom you must work. Like the surgeon, your radiologist should have board certification and advanced training in the treatment of cancer. That means the radiologist has completed a hospital course of training in radiology and has passed an examination of skill and competence in that field. Additionally, he or she has studied the precise treatment of cancer with radiation and has fulfilled all of the requirements for certification in that field as well. Once you are certain of the radiologist's credentials, obtain personal recommendations from hospital colleagues and assistants who are familiar with the doctor's techniques and reputation.

Oncologists

The third type of standard cancer therapy is chemotherapy. It involves the use of anticancer drugs administered by a medical oncologist or a hematologist with oncology training. The medical oncologist treats all forms of cancer with the appropriate chemotherapeutic agents. The hematologist usually treats cancers of the blood, such as leukemia and lymphoma, but can treat other forms of cancer as well. Be sure board certification and extensive experience are part of the credentials of the oncologist recommended to you, and make certain that he or she has dealt with cases similar to yours. This assures you that you have selected the best doctor for your treatment.

Having sought out and secured excellent medical or surgical professionals, you are well on your way to a successful recovery. You can feel confident that you are in the best hands. But this is just the start. Your treatment has another important component.

A FABULOUS FINISH

If you had to win a one-mile race to save your life and had to compete against the finest world-class milers in existence today, you would probably lose the race and lose your life. But if you could start fifty yards from the finish line, and all the other runners had to begin at the starting line, you would probably win the race and save your life. Well, you can place yourself within winning distance of the finish line by securing the finest doctors available to work on your case. If that means traveling to receive your health care or inconveniencing yourself to get the best, then so be it. Remember, a great start sets the pace for a great finish.

Still, you must go the extra fifty yards to win the race. Even with the best surgical or medical help you can find, your cure is not guaranteed. In fact, your doctor will usually say, "I *think* you'll be all right; I *think* we got it all." Unfortunately, that's just not good enough. If even a small piece of the tumor is left behind, if just a few cells escape removal or eradication, your troubles may return. So take the steps that increase your chances of complete success and total cure. To truly win the race, you must actually cross the finish line, you must go the extra distance yourself. You can do this through the use of the adjunct therapies described in this book.

A WORD ABOUT CONFLICTING OPINIONS

In general the treatments of most cancers are standardized and reflect what have been statistically the most successful approaches to cancer, thus providing you with the greatest chances of being cured. A good doctor will tell you about these statistically preferred treatments, furnish you with realistic alternatives, if they exist, and then make a recommendation. Of course, physicians have differences of opinion in certain cases, but if you are dealing with the finest doctors in the profession, you will get the best care, no matter what approach you decide to take. Many times, you will have to make the final treatment decision *yourself*. Educate yourself as much as possible so that you can make intelligent choices. Where two experts have significantly divergent opinions, you must seek a third consultant.

There might also be a difference of opinion between your traditional doctors and the adjunct therapists and physicians you come to work with. My recommendation is to follow the traditional doctor's advice as it relates to his or her specialty and to uphold the adjunct physician's counsel as it pertains to that person's treatments. Each has an expertise in a specific area and should intelligently limit his or her individual influence to that area of expertise. If a physician or other therapist *insists* that you listen only to him or her, look for a replacement. Remember: It's your body and your life!

Recommended Reading

American Medical Directory. 28th ed. 4 vol. Chicago: American Medical Association, 1982.

Auerbach, M. and T. Bogue. *Getting Yours: A Consumer's Guide to Obtaining Your Medical Records.* Washington, DC: Public Citizens Health Research Group, 1978.

Berman, H., D. Burhenne, and L. Rose. *The Complete Health Care Advisor.* New York: St. Martin's Press, 1983.

Breslow, L., ed. *How to Get the Best Health Care for Your Money.* Emmaus, PA: Rodale, 1977.

Crile, G. Jr. *Surgery: Your Choices, Your Alternatives.* New York: Delacorte, 1978.

Directory of Medical Specialists. 21st ed. 2 vol. Chicago: Marquis, 1983.

Eiseman, B. *What Are My Chances?* Philadelphia: Saunders, 1980.

Lehrer, S. *Alternative Treatments for Cancer.* Chicago: Nelson-Hall, 1979.

Lemaitre, G. D. *How to Choose a Good Doctor.* Andover, MA: Andover Publishing Group, 1979.

Morra, M. and E. Potts. *Choices: Realistic Alternatives in Cancer Treatments.* New York: Avon, 1980.

Pekkanen, J. *The Best Doctors in the U.S.* New York: Seaview, 1981.

Rosenfeld, I. *Second Opinion: Your Medical Alternatives.* New York: Bantam, 1981.

Salsbury, K. H., and E. L. Johnson. *The Indispensable Cancer Handbook: A Comprehensive, Authoritative Guide to the Latest and Best in Diagnosis, Treatment, Care, and Supportive Services.* New York: Wideview, 1981.

4
What You Need to Know About Cancer

To appreciate the nature of the therapies in this book and to maximize their benefits, you should first understand a few things about the disease you're going to conquer. This is not an easy task, however, because cancer is a complicated and confusing problem. It has been described as a wide variety of illnesses, with many causes and numerous effects on different areas of the body. Cancer can act differently in different people, and treatments can vary from one institution to another. Not even experts fully agree on the nature of the disease, and they often cite various definitions, causes, patterns, and even different names for identical forms of the same illness.

Perhaps the easiest way to understand the disease is to realize that all tumors represent new or recent cell growth. They are the manifestation of cells that have literally gone crazy, embarking on a meaningless mission of unlimited multiplication. They develop and expand haphazardly—without restriction—and in total violation of the normal boundaries of adjacent tissues and organs.

In addition, there seems to be no purpose to the cellular arrangement of the tumor. Unlike liver or kidney cells, for instance, which assume an exact configuration to perform certain functions for the body, tumor cells grow wildly and spread indiscriminately wherever they please. They live only to divide and disperse in total disregard of their surroundings.

FROM ONE CELL, AN ENTIRE TUMOR

As the original tumor cell grows and divides, it generates two new cells similar to itself. These two then rapidly divide, forming four similar cells, and so on. The cell reproduction continues and with each division, the resultant cells become increasingly abnormal. Eventually, this process creates a small mass of abnormal cells—the tumor—which begins to displace or destroy the normal cells from which it originated.

BENIGN VS. MALIGNANT

By studying the tumor, doctors can determine whether it is benign or malignant. Benign means that it will not endanger life, unless it is situated in a vital area such as the brain. Generally, benign tumors grow slowly, pushing aside the surrounding normal tissue as they expand. Unlike malignant tumors, benign tumors do not infiltrate or grow between normal cells, nor do they travel to distant parts of the body. Instead, they remain where they begin, growing slowly in a confined area.

Malignant tumors, on the other hand, endanger life as their growth continues unhindered. Usually they grow rapidly and quickly invade surrounding areas, destroying everything in their path. They spread (metastasize) to other areas of the body by moving into blood vessels and entering the bloodstream or by penetrating lymph channels and migrating to regional lymph glands. Wherever they come to rest—in the lungs, liver, or brain, for example—they implant themselves and start another colony of similar tumor cells. The same process of cell division that produced the primary tumor forms secondary tumors (metastases). These will behave in the same way as the primary tumor, expanding locally, destroying surrounding normal tissue, encroaching into and eroding blood vessels and lymph channels and extending to even more distant regions of the body. The malignant tumor is the type referred to as cancer.

CANCER

To gain an even more intimate understanding of the differences between normal and cancerous cells, imag-

Figure A
NORMAL CELL

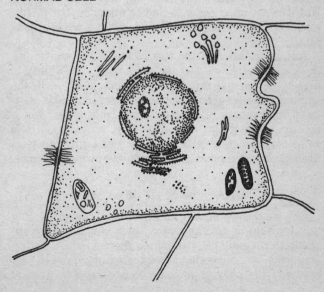

ine you are looking through a microscope at two exemplary cells magnified 32,000 times life size. First, look at the normal cell in Figure A. This is a well-organized cell. It borders smoothly with its neighbors and is regular and symmetrical. The cell's brain, its nucleus, is round and regular, and its genetic material, chromatin, is fine and uniform. Within the nucleus, the genes that control all cell functions are working perfectly, directing the production of DNA and RNA soon to be passed to the awaiting protein producers, the ribosomes.

Now take a look at the cancer cell in Figure B. Instead of one nucleus, it has two. The larger of the two is irregular in size, shape, and consistency. The chromatin within this nucleus is coarse and clumped together in jagged masses. Compare this irregular nucleus to the nucleus of the normal cell. In addition to the larger nucleus, there is a smaller, denser one. It, too, is totally abnormal and incapable of directing the cell to perform any normal task. Not all cancer cells have two nuclei as depicted in the drawing. Most have only one. But it is not uncommon to find as many as four or five nuclei within one cancer cell, and at times no nucleus at all.

An examination of the rest of the cell reveals other irregularities. Since the nucleus has lost the ability to direct the normal internal operations of the cell, the small organelles are no longer present. Instead, the cytoplasm is empty, except for small void areas, which contain nothing and have absolutely no function. The cell's only function is to reproduce and grow in total disregard of the surrounding cells, tissues, and organs.

DNA: The Stuff of Genes

How do these mutated, cancerous cells develop? Why do they reproduce unhindered in a way that is traumatic to the very body in which they exist? To understand the principles that allow the natural growth processes in the body to go completely awry, you need to

Figure B
CANCER CELL

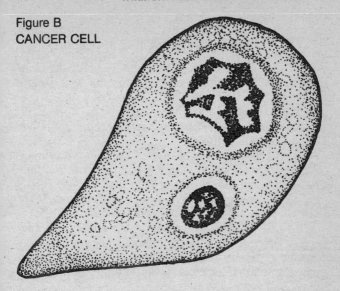

comprehend the functioning of life's most basic and essential blueprint: DNA. These three letters, which stand for deoxyribonucleic acid, the molecular basis of heredity (genes), tell the entire story and explain the ultimate cause of cancer. To uncover their secrets, you must increase the power of your imaginary microscope to 150,000 times life size and see what new universes await deep within the cell nucleus.

As you magnify and focus on a single cell, aiming at its center, your microscope brings you to the cell nucleus, then projects you down into the chromatin that composes the nucleus and farther into the genes themselves. Deeper still, you encounter the substance that actually makes up your genes, the DNA, and finally you can see its true chemical structure, consisting of organic bases, phosphates, and sugars.

Two doctors, James Watson and Francis Crick, first established the exact physical structure of DNA in 1953 and described its spiral-staircase structure, shown in

Figure C. DNA is essentially composed of two swirling ribbons of chemical compounds linked together by sub-microscopic atomic bridges called hydrogen bonds. Each strand is perfectly paired with its exact chemical mate to create a living chemical computer that directs the performance of every cell in the body and determines individual human characteristics. All human life is created and directed by the chemical chains of DNA and the genes it contains.

Just as there are genes that control height and eye color, there are also genes that determine how fast cells grow and when they will reproduce and divide. This is precisely where cancer originates—in the segments of DNA that control growth and reproduction.

With just a minor alteration in the chemical structure of DNA, a cell's entire existence is modified because its genetic material is changed. With this change come a multitude of consequences, some minor, some major, and some devastating.

If, for instance, the change destroys a gene that directs the production of a single compound in just one cell in just one area of the liver, no great damage is done, since literally millions of other cells are ready and able to carry on the work. The loss of a single cell is trivial. If, on the other hand, the change affects a gene that controls cell growth and reproduction, the effects could be far-reaching. The mutated cell may start to grow wildly, dividing unnaturally and without purpose. This process creates a tumor cell, which goes on to produce a group of similarly mutated cells that will continue to reproduce uncontrollably, passing on the mutated genes to all resultant cells. Eventually a whole colony of mutated cells develops and becomes what is known as a tumor. Thus, the cause of cancer is actually a chemical change, a mutation, that occurs in the DNA of just one cell.

To clarify these thoughts, look for a moment at the example of skin cancer, or squamous carcinoma of the

**Figure C
DNA**

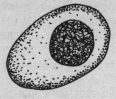

Living Cell

DNA is found within
the genes in the nucleus
of the cell.

DNA

Its ribbonlike structure is
composed of specific
chemical compounds that
are arranged in a special
order.

Atomic Structure

When just one of these
compounds is changed and
the special arrangement is
altered, a genetic mutation
occurs, and this can lead to
cancer.

skin. This type of cancer is caused by chronic overexpo-
sure to sunlight and often occurs in individuals with

fair skin and light hair. As the sun's ultraviolet rays bombard and penetrate the sensitive skin, day after day, year after year, they slowly take their toll on the skin in the form of chronic burning, irritation, and degeneration. This ongoing process destroys millions upon millions of skin cells, which are replaced by normal, healthy cells, which are then themselves destroyed as the harmful exposure continues.

While the initial skin changes are superficial, affecting just the more durable outer layers of cells, continued exposure causes ultraviolet light to extend into deeper, more sensitive tissues and, ultimately, to reach the fragile immature cells that were once protected by the older outer cells. Like miniature laser beams, the ultraviolet rays bombard everything in their path, striking cell after cell, killing or damaging the younger internal cells while releasing dangerous light energy into the skin.

While some cells manage to escape with only minor injury, repair themselves, and survive, others are irreversibly altered so that they cannot possibly undergo repair or return to normal functioning. Instead, they are permanently mutated—alive but abnormal, unpredictable, and uncontrollable. In their nuclei, which have been battered by countless rays, the DNA is critically altered, and the genes that control cell growth and reproduction are permanently modified. Now, released from the normal constraints of reproduction and division, these mutated cells are free to reproduce at will and can go on to produce an isolated colony of clones, which will eventually enlarge into a tumor.

Of course, this is only one example, but the principle is universal: Genetic mutations are the real cause of cancer. In this particular case, the genetic mutation (the DNA alteration) is caused by the ultraviolet rays of the sun, but the causative agent can vary. It may be a toxin in cigarette smoke that causes lung cancer, or additives in food that cause colon cancer. It could be dioxin in the drinking water or radiation from a toxic spill. Regardless, the ultimate cause of cancer is the chromosomal damage within the cell nucleus—the DNA mutation that releases a cell from its normal growth and reproductive process and converts it into a malignant cell that generates a tumor.

CARCINOGENS, INITIATORS, AND PROMOTERS

Now that you have seen how mutations in the DNA cause the unhindered generation and growth of tumors, the next step is to identify what causes these deadly mutations. As you doubtless already know, many substances cause cancer. These *carcinogens*, as they are called, abound throughout nature. Some are naturally occurring, like the ultraviolet rays of the sun, while others are of human origin, like the radioactive contamination from nuclear accidents such as the one at Chernobyl. Regardless of a carcinogen's nature or origin, its effects can be disastrous to human life if exposure is extreme or prolonged.

Generally it takes more than just a single carcinogen to permanently alter DNA and produce a tumor. Usually another substance or group of harmful agents is required. These secondary factors, are called promoters, and they bring the carcinogen to its full potential. In other words, *carcinogens* initiate the tumor process by converting a normal cell into a malignant cell. Thus, they can also be called *initiators*. To produce their malignant effects, they usually require the aid of other substances, called *promoters*, which *promote* the growth of cancer.

Occasionally, if the exposure to a carcinogen is extremely high, no promoter is needed to start tumor growth. But more often the various harmful agents work together. Consider the following experiment as an example of documented proof of the process of initiation and promotion. Scientists used laboratory test mice as subjects in this investigation. First, the researchers exposed the mice's skin to a relatively low dose of benzopyrene, a known carcinogen. Nothing happened. Then, croton oil, which is *not* carcinogenic, was painted on the same areas of skin that had been exposed to benzopyrene, and tumors soon grew abundantly. The carcinogen benzopyrene *initiated* the tumor formation, but it was not until croton oil, the *promoter*, was applied that a tumor formed. If croton oil alone were painted on the skin or applied before the benzopyrene, no tumor growth was noted. The lethal combination was benzopyrene initiation followed by croton oil. Similarly, a common barbiturate, phenobarbitol, promotes tumors in the liver following exposure to diethylnitrosamine. Saccharin will stimulate lung cancer growth after a single initiation by urethane.

Numerous articles have been written on the subject of initiators and promoters, citing hundreds of deadly associations. In each case, the step-by-step process may be slightly different, but the general principle is the same. Carcinogenesis is a multistage process and usually involves more than simply the exposure to a single carcinogenic agent.

This concept of initiation and promotion is important in understanding the general causes of cancer, but more specifically it helps to explain why cancer may selectively strike one person and not another, even when individual exposure to a carcinogenic agent seems equal. A promoter is needed to activate the carcinogen, and that promoter may be unique to the individual.

Additionally, the promotion of cancer may come from substances manufactured and liberated by the body— harmful chemicals and hormones that prevent the body's natural defenses from operating normally. These chemicals result from a disharmony between the mind and the body. They are the products of frustration and discontent. They are the natural consequence of our stressful existence.

But all of these problems, along with the subsequent development of cancer, have been anticipated. In our creation, we were given a vast array of defense mechanisms, a virtual arsenal of protection to safeguard us from our natural enemies and even from ourselves. In constant battles occurring within our bodies, the forces of our immune systems fight the harmful germs that cause infections and the malignant cells that compose tumors. Each agent of the "bad system" has enemies in the "good system," designed specifically to identify, attack, and eliminate them when they appear. As part of the "good system," the cells and substances of the natural defense system form an intricate check-and-balance network that prevents or reverses disease and can identify and eliminate cancer.

5
The Natural Defense System

Every hour, every minute, every second of your life, cellular wars are fought within your body. Your body fights off disease, viruses, and cancer many times without your even knowing it, for the battles occur on a tiny, cellular scale. Just as you are often exposed to bacteria and viruses and do not get sick, your body "gets" cancer (contains cancerous cells) many times, and your natural defense system identifies, destroys, and eliminates the malignant cells swiftly and completely.

Many of the body's cancer-fighting substances have been discovered, and scientists will soon uncover many more as they probe ever deeper into the secrets of the body's natural defense system. This chapter will lead you on a tour of this natural defense system and introduce you to some of the many cells and chemicals that compose it. They are vital to preventing and curing cancer. The best news is that we all produce these substances if our natural defense system is in good shape.

But what if the natural defense system is not healthy,

if it has allowed a malignant tumor to begin and grow? Exposure to carcinogens, as discussed in the previous chapter, may have punched holes in the body's natural defense system. Physical and mental forces may have contributed to the system's breakdown. (You'll discover more about these forces in later chapters.) But the natural defense system does not have to remain permanently weakened! As you saw in Chapters 2 and 3, it can be reactivated. Regenerating and strengthening this system is within your power; it is what you must do to be well again.

To do this, you must believe in your body's power to heal itself. You must truly understand that your defenses against cancer are not pipe dreams or flukes, but concrete, marvelous parts of your natural makeup, created to keep or get you well. By knowing the basics about your body's cancer-fighting agents, you will be better armed mentally and emotionally to activate them for your health.

THE AMAZING STORY OF INTERFERON

Perhaps you have heard or read about the substance *interferon* and its ability to fight cancer. It is probably the most widely studied and publicized of the substances known to promote the remission of this disease. It is just one of the many anticancer agents produced by the human body, but its fascinating story reveals how wonderfully the natural defense system works—and can be set to work within you.

The road leading to interferon's discovery was complicated and time-consuming, spanning more than 150 years. The travelers were a multitude of doctors and researchers, beginning with Edward Jenner as long ago as 1805. There were too many experiments to mention fully here, but two distinct milestones guided those who would walk in Jenner's footsteps.

The first occurred in 1937, when two astute British

researchers, Drs. Findley and MacCallum, noted that monkeys infected with Raft Valley fever virus were somehow protected from the subsequent infection and fatal effects of yellow fever virus. As reported by Alick Isaacs in *Scientific American* those two scientists coined the phrase "viral interference" and postulated that when one virus infects a group of cells, a second virus is somehow excluded.

They further presumed, and other scientists concurred, that viral interference could take place within the human body as well. Clinical proof of this, the second milestone, was noted in the mid-1950s, when Mexican children were given oral polio vaccine but failed to develop antibodies against the polio virus. In the normal chain of events, the vaccine, a weakened form of the polio virus, would cause a mild infection in the intestine and stimulate the production of antipolio antibodies. But in the Mexican children, this just didn't happen. Instead, all the children harbored a second virus, a common intestinal variety, which interfered with the polio virus and prevented the development of immunity.

The Breakthrough

For a number of years, the actual cause of this viral interference remained unknown. How could the presence of one virus prevent an infection by a second? Then in 1957, Jean Lindermann and Alick Isaacs from the National Institute of Medical Research in England made an important discovery. They found that a few hours after they treated a living cell culture with a dead virus, the culture medium (the fluid that bathed the living cells) could interfere with a secondary viral infection. When fresh cells were added to the medium, they were somehow protected by an antiviral substance that had been released into the fluid. With this knowledge, Drs. Isaacs and Lindermann eventually isolated and then identified the mysterious antiviral substance. They called it interferon.

Many more experiments were performed after 1957, and many properties in addition to viral interference were attributed to interferon. Most importantly, the substance was shown to exhibit strong anticancer effects.

Because of interferon's ability to cause viral interference, researchers reasoned that it could also limit the potentially deadly infections of cancer-causing viruses and thereby prevent cancers from developing. Scientists soon demonstrated that interferon could prevent the intracellular multiplication of cancer viruses and also block the transformation of a viral infected cell into a tumor cell. This observation was made several times from 1961 through 1969 by noted authorities around the world. With these new findings, interest grew, and experimentation continued at a furious pace. More far-reaching discoveries were made.

A delay or reversal in tumor growth was observed in laboratory animals after they were exposed to certain viruses. Although it was initially thought that the virus itself attacked and killed the animal's cancer, this theory was quickly dismissed, and interferon emerged as the anticancer agent.

Two researchers, D. P. Atanasiu and C. Chany, showed that injection of hamsters with a moderately pure extract of interferon twenty-four hours before inoculation with lethal polyoma virus not only delayed the appearance of tumors, reduced the number of tumors, and augmented the animal survival rate, but also increased the number of tumor-free animals. When tumors were transplanted from one animal to another, injections of interferon likewise inhibited the tumor growth. Here was solid evidence that real antitumor, not just antiviral, activity was attributable to interferon.

The data on interferon were becoming more and more complex. As new information poured in, the wonders of this new "drug" revealed themselves in a wide variety of ways, and the scope of interferon's effect on viruses and cancer broadened with each passing day. Still, the next question loomed great in the minds of everyone involved in the interferon story: What about humans? Sure, laboratory experiments with test tubes and hamsters seemed promising, but would interferon hold its clout where it really counted? So the next step was human trials.

Dusseldorf, Germany, 1981

A five-year-old girl who suffered from recurrent papillomatosis of the larynx was requiring continuous surgical removal of the mushroomlike tumors that grew in her voice box around her vocal cords every three to four weeks. Her condition gradually worsened until she finally required an emergency tracheotomy, a life-saving procedure, in order to allow her to breathe. Rapid and extensive spread of the tumor had packed her entire larynx and upper trachea with tumor cells, preventing air from reaching her lungs.

In a desperate search for new and lasting therapy, the doctors initiated treatment with interferon, first intravenously, then subcutaneously, at a rate of 2 million international units (IU) per day. In only four weeks, the formerly extensive and life-threatening papillomatosis was significantly reduced. The doctors made a second surprising observation. If the dosage of interferon was halved, the tumors began to reappear. But if the dose was increased to 2 million IU, the new growth could be repressed, indicating a relationship between the amount of interferon administered and the success of the treatment.

Helsinki, Finland, 1981

In an almost identical case, for two and a half years a young boy had been treated surgically for recurrent papillomatosis of the larynx. Explosive growth of the tumor necessitated an emergency tracheotomy to preserve the child's life. And again, in a final attempt to save the boy, interferon injections were initiated. As in the previous case, within four weeks of receiving the interferon, the child was miraculously improved. But unlike the first case, the tumors not only reduced in size and number, they totally disappeared.

Zagreb, Yugoslavia, 1981

The patient was a forty-nine-year-old man referred to University Hospital in Zagreb for a growth in the back of the throat, overlying the right tonsil. A biopsy was performed, and the diagnosis of squamous carcinoma was made from the biopsy material. Immediate treatment with interferon began with injections around the tumor nodule and along the base of the tongue.

During the course of therapy, the tumor nodule shrank, eventually flattened out, and became indistinguishable from the surrounding tissue. In addition, a shallow ulcer in the center of the tumor first sealed over with a whitish deposit, then healed completely and was absorbed into the adjacent tissue of the throat.

At this point in the therapy, the area where the tumor had been located was surgically removed and examined under a microscope. In the region of the tumor base, only scar tissue and inflammatory cells could be seen. No cancer cells were present. In the area at the base of the tongue, enlargement of the lymph gland was noted, but no cancer cells were seen. And local lymph nodes revealed no evidence of tumors whatsoever. Instead, they showed a strong immune reaction, indicating a positive natural defense response. In just three months, the patient was completely cured of his disease.

These are just three isolated cases from the annals of medical science. Yet they provide amazing evidence of interferon's ability to arrest or reverse tumor growth in

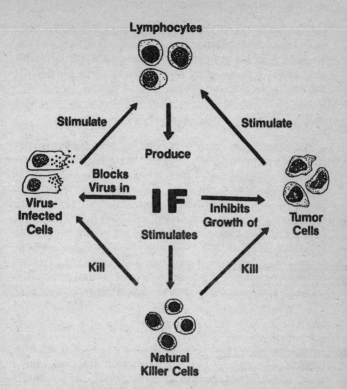

THE EFFECTS OF INTERFERON (IF)*

Virus, virus-infected cells, and tumor cells stimulate lymphocytes to make interferon. Interferon then transforms other lymphocytes into natural killer cells, limits the growth of tumor cells, or blocks viral infection of other cells. Natural killer cells go on to destroy either virus-infected cells or tumor cells.

*Adapted from "Mechanism of Activation of Human Natural Killer Cells Against Tumors" by Daniela Santori and Hilary Koprowski. *Immunological Review.* Vol. 44, 1979: 155. Used with permission of the publisher, Munksgaard International Publishers, Ltd., Copenhagen, Denmark. Copyright © 1979.

human subjects. And that itself is wonderful news. Still, the most amazing fact about interferon and all the other wonderful anticancer cells and substances is that they are all produced by each and every one of us. They are all manufactured by the human body!

YOUR ARMY OF NATURAL DEFENDERS

You have a vast array of cancer fighters at your disposal. They are intricately interconnected, and they have so many sources and functions that there is too little room to discuss them here. Yet their very existence proves that your body wants to stay healthy. The following descriptions are simplified, and they do not begin to include all the biological substances and functions that fight cancer. But they will give you a valuable and encouraging picture of how your body's natural cancer fighters can work together to help you cure yourself—without your help or your even knowing it.

Cancer Identifiers

Imagine a part of your body—perhaps a kidney or a lung. Each day as it performs its given function, maintaining your health and life, new cells are created within it, old cells die, and foreign substances may try to enter it and are rendered harmless and destroyed. But what happens when this natural sequence is broken, when the natural chemical balance is disturbed and a mutated cell appears? Your body has many substances that identify cancer cells and can thus start the processes that will destroy them.

Among the most important are the *monocytes*. These white blood cells circulate through your bloodstream and can identify bacteria, viruses, or malignant cells. If they discover any abnormal cells, they can enter body tissues and convert into specialized fighting cells called *macrophages*. Sometimes the macrophages themselves are the first to identify cancer; they're always wandering through the body's tissues on the lookout. If the macrophages spot cancer, they stimulate T lymphocytes to "call out the troops." Like monocytes, *T lymphocytes* are a type of white blood cell, but unlike monocytes, they can convert to plasma cells, which in turn create antibodies.

Antibodies not only find cancer cells but attach themselves to the cell walls. They then attract their *complements*, which perform a variety of defense activities. Activated by the antibodies, the nine kinds of complements perform their assigned tasks, from punching holes in cancer cell walls to tagging the malignant opponent so that other cancer fighters can identify it more easily. The process of destruction has begun.

Cancer Killers

Perhaps the most awesome members of the natural defense system are the natural killer cells, so named for their ability to liquify their malignant opponents. In 1978, researchers discovered that these killer cells are a specialized type of T lymphocyte solely devoted to slaying tumor cells. Their method is to manufacture a host of caustic substances that literally break down the structure of cancer.

The killer cells' arsenal includes *superoxide* and *hydrogen peroxide*, both of which fizz away cancer cells, just as the household version of hydrogen peroxide bubbles away the impurities in a cut or wound. *Lysolecithin* acts like a heavy-duty detergent taking wax off a table, weakening tumor cell walls by stripping off their protection. *Protease* and *phospholipase* eat away the cell walls themselves. They also produce *lymphotoxin*, a toxic chemical that actually poisons the weakened malignant cells.

An additional anticancer substance called *tumor necrosis factor* (TNF) has recently been discovered and shown to decompose tumor masses. Researchers all over the world are experimenting with this substance, trying to manufacture enough of it synthetically to administer to cancer patients who seem unable to generate the proper amount for themselves. TNF has been shown to cause tumor delay within twenty-four hours of administration, and hopes are high that TNF will soon be commercially available. But remember, too, TNF is created naturally by the human body!

Another key to spontaneous remission is the process called *phagocytosis*. One cell that destroys cancer by this method is the mighty macrophage. Macrophages and their counterparts, monocytes, actively search the body for active cancer cells, faithfully awaiting the first sign of trouble. If they find cancer, a complex series of interactions transforms them into phagocytes. By traveling in the bloodstream, they quickly migrate to the sinister tumor mass and surround it. One by one, they wiggle and squeeze between the separate tumor cells and gradually make their way to the heart of the tumor mass. Finally, like individual warriors, each macrophage singles out a specific opponent and embraces it in a struggle to the death, surrounding it, engulfing it, and ultimately incorporating it into its body.

Once malignant cells have been engulfed (phagocytized), a second, more critical series of events begins to unfold. The imprisoned cells start to degenerate. Their bodies begin to shrink, and their cellular contents liquify. Eventually they are reduced to small, dark, round masses, which ultimately disappear from inside the bodies of the ferocious macrophages.

Antispread Agents

While natural killer cells attack and destroy cancer, other substances prevent its spread. The antiviral chemical interferon, as discussed earlier, effectively curbs the growth of cancer by preventing the viral mutations that cause cancer cells in the first place. Its presence in the body also prevents cancer cells from migrating, and it slows their reproduction. As you saw in the case studies described earlier, it also stimulates the natural killer cells to peak activity.

The body also produces a substance called *interleukin*, which similarly prevents cancer's spread. Scientists are still working to find out exactly how it operates but already know that it interferes with the metabolism of cancer cells. It has already proved useful in producing cancer regression in laboratory experiments. Continuing research will uncover more about interleukin's potential. One thing is certain: Interleukin is one more link in a system designed to choke the spread and growth of cancer.

Cancer Eliminators

Once cancer cells are killed, either by natural killer cells or through phagocytosis, they are completely removed from the body. Macrophages, after engulfing and eating cancer cells in the process of phagocytosis, digest them and self-destruct. The body eliminates the remains through the intestines or spleen. Cancer destroyed by other means is eliminated by granulocytes, a type of white blood cell. They consume the leftover pieces of dead cancer cells and, like macrophages, self-destruct and are carried away through the body's natural elimination processes.

It is wonderful to contemplate how completely and thoroughly our bodies can rid themselves of cancer! From the identification of a malignant growth to the final sloughing off of dead cancer cells, each step is part of an intricate, powerful system. Perhaps even more powerful is our power to influence it.

KEEPING YOUR NATURAL DEFENSE SYSTEM IN SHAPE

While the natural defense system is a sophisticated network of cells and substances that protect the body against disease, it is also vulnerable to a wide variety of elements and conditions that can either weaken or strengthen it. Its effectiveness is intimately associated with each person's genetic makeup, physical condition, and lifestyle, and its integrity can literally change from day to day, perhaps even hour to hour.

Age

One force that constantly works against us is aging. From puberty on, the thymus gland, a small organ of immunity in the neck, begins to shrink. While this change is not outwardly noticeable, its internal ramifications are dramatic. Because the thymus is the origin of vital T lymphocytes, its reduction and gradual disappearance by age 60 means that the number of competent natural defense cells also diminishes. Since the ability to fight off disease depends on the quantity and quality of lymph cells, the body gradually becomes more susceptible to illness and to diseases like cancer.

Stress

Besides the aging process, which is continuous, several temporary states adversely affect the immune response. One of them is stress, a psychological condition with many physical side effects. Although the natural human reactions to stressful situations are essential to survival, prolonged stress levies a heavy toll on the entire body. It affects the function of all the body's organs and systems, including the natural defense system. The insidious action of prolonged steroid release all but shuts down the immune system, and the enemies of the body—the bacteria, the viruses, and the cancer cells that are normally held in check—have a golden opportunity to run wild. Fortunately, the ill effects of stress can be controlled, and the techniques used to manage stress effectively are virtually the same as those that bolster the immune system and inhibit the growth and spread of cancer.

Cigarettes and Alcohol

Two habits that are established health risks are smoking and drinking. Health experts have called them to our attention time and time again, and the Surgeon General has beseeched us to reduce alcohol consumption and to abandon smoking completely. True, both of these activities are associated with specific forms of cancer; but they also affect us in ways that are much less obvious. Excessive alcohol consumption has been shown to depress the inflammatory response, a basic function of the immune system, and heavy cigarette smoking significantly alters the proportion of lymphocytes in the white blood cell count. Overall, the general incidence of cancer is higher among smokers and drinkers, and several investigators cite alterations in the natural defense system as the probable cause.

Nutrition

Nutrition is also connected to the competence of the immune system. In remote parts of the world, where children suffer from rampant malnutrition, they also experience much higher rates of infection and problems with their immune response to illness. In relation to cancer, iron, zinc, and vitamin C seem to be the critical dietary elements, along with the essential and nonessential amino acids—the building blocks of protein. In-depth blood analyses show that a lack of these nutrients is linked with a reduction in the number of T lymphocytes and a greatly compromised thymus gland. To further complicate the picture, it now appears likely that even small deficiencies in critical vitamins and minerals might be sufficient to alter the natural defense system enough to compromise its function and allow the growth of cancer.

Fatty Foods

As surprising as it may be, fatty foods have a deleterious effect on the natural defense system. It is the fat, pure and simple, that is the culprit. Studies conducted on laboratory animals have established a direct connection between premature aging and excessive amounts of fat in the diet. Measurable deficiencies in the immune system and in immune cells also have been noted. Recent studies from the National Cancer Institute have demonstrated an astonishing correlation between high-fat diets and the development of cancer—a full 35 percent of cancer cases are attributed to low-fiber and high-fat diets. Apparently, fatty foods stimulate the secretion of bile and steroids into the intestines, causing excessive wear and tear on intestinal cells. In some way, this causes a subsequent reduction in the effectiveness of the immune system.

REVIVING A WEAKENED NATURAL DEFENSE SYSTEM

The factors described here are only some of the causes of a weakened defense system and an increased susceptibility to cancer. There are many others, ranging from chemicals found in contaminated drinking water to the virus that causes AIDS. These elements must be completely avoided in order to ensure good health. Other negative factors, like the ones we have discussed, can be modified, and the natural defense system can be restored to optimal performance. In other words, while we have little control over the carcinogens (initiators), we stand a good chance of controlling our internal promoters. And this alone can make a huge difference.

For example, while age constantly works against us, scientists have uncovered methods for at least slowing down the aging process. Certain substances, specifically the antioxidants that are occasionally used as food preservatives, appear to preserve our youth as well as our food. In fact, in countries where the use of these substances is uncommon, the rate of certain cancers is higher. This is not to say that we should make a habit of eating preservatives, though they do appear to slow aging. It does suggest, however, that healthy antioxidants, including vitamin E and selenium, can be important in the avoidance and cure of certain cancers. Potassium, too, seems to preserve the integrity of our cells and possibly prevents the unkind effects of aging at the cellular level. Vitamins have their place also, since they appear to forestall many of the diseases attributable to the aging process.

Poor habits like drinking and smoking can generally be broken—returning a previously depressed natural defense system to normal function. Dietary corrections can halt the detrimental effects of excess fat or too little protein. Interestingly, specific dietary programs and vitamin supplementations can stimulate the entire immune system, bringing it to a level of supercompetence and amazing effectiveness.

Daily aerobic exercise has also been shown to bolster general health and the power of the natural defense system. In ways not fully understood, better conditioning improves all internal functions, and the immune system performs more efficiently. Perhaps this is due to an increased oxygenation of all tissues, including the bone marrow and the lymph glands, or maybe it is related to the reduction of stress and the subsequent liberation of the immune system to perform better. Regardless, its effects are real and certainly beneficial.

From what you now know about the development of cancer and the natural defense system's role in keeping cancer in check, you should understand the importance of maintaining a healthy immune system. You should also realize that your illness is an indication that somewhere, somehow, your immune system weakened and allowed one malignant cell to escape detection and progress into a full-grown tumor. Although this was a critical faltering, it is not irreversible. The studies of miraculous spontaneous remissions show that the immune system is resilient, that in the face of adversity, it can bounce back with amazing force and speed to once again take control and eliminate the malignancy. Through the action of anticancer substances regularly produced by the body—from the superoxide that literally fizzes away cancer cells to the tumor necrosis factor that melts away tumors like butter on a hot stove—you can arrest the cancer growth and restore yourself to good health.

A big part of keeping your natural defense system in shape is making sure that your mind is not sabotaging your body. Every year, scientists find new ways in which our thoughts and actions affect how we feel. From these discoveries, it now appears that stress is, indeed, a major factor in the body's health. The next chapter will clarify the connection between stress and health; introduce you to some miraculous, curative substances that your body produces when you're happy; and give you more tools to use in reversing the negative forces in your body and unleashing the good ones.

6
The Link Between the Mind and the Body

In Chapter 5 you learned one of the reasons why cancer may selectively strike one person and not another, even though each individual's exposure to the carcinogenic agent seems equal. You saw how personal susceptibility is increased by cancer initiators and promoters working together. Yet other basic and natural factors can increase an individual's chances of growing a tumor. You may be surprised to know that these factors are more psychological than physical, relating to anxiety, emotional conflict, and the mind's effect on the body.

AVOIDING THE BAD SYSTEM

Under normal circumstances, cancer cannot develop within our bodies because of our built-in natural defense mechanisms. Rapid identification and swift elimination of any malignant cells keep us healthy and cancer-free. That's the job of the immune system and its cancer-surveillance function. Whenever cancer does oc-

cur, it results from a failure of the body's natural defenses, a breakdown in the immune system, and the
creation of a negative internal environment that supports the growth of malignant cells. I refer to this as the
"BAD SYSTEM," and it is intricately related to the
psychological and physical effects of stress.

Of course, we all expect to experience a certain
amount of tension and anxiety. But when the strain
becomes too great, it can have a strong effect on our
physical well-being. Perhaps you have heard of people
who have suffered misfortune and then poor health, of a
man who lost his wife and shortly thereafter died of
lung cancer, of a woman who developed uterine cancer
when her youngest child left home for good. Stories like
these abound and compose the case studies of medical
researchers who investigate the relationship between
the mind and the body.

But how does the mind so influence the body? How is
it that emotional and psychological conflicts can lead to
the growth of a malignant tumor? To answer these
questions, we must address the subjects of brain function and immunity to disease—two aspects of the link
between the mind and the body.

The Brain's Role in Maintaining
the Immune System

The human brain is divided into two major parts, the
upper brain (*cortex*) and the lower brain (*subcortex*). In
the upper brain, higher mental function occurs and
sensation and movement originate. Furthermore, this
is the site of all intellectual activity. This activity includes reading and language comprehension, memory,
judgment, and intellectual abstraction. Through the action of the cortex, we are made aware of our environment, interact with our surroundings, and relate to
reality.

The activities of the lower brain, though nonintellectual, hold equally important functions. For instance, an important component of the lower brain is the limbic system. More than just a specific structure or location, it is actually a group of interconnecting tracts that link independent sections of the brain and allow the cortex to communicate with the subcortex. This part of the lower brain is concerned with emotions and behavior and provides an outlet for expressing feelings. The limbic system also records mental stress, translates it into specific feelings like depression and despair, and transmits this information to other parts of the brain, specifically the hypothalamus.

The *hypothalamus*, a small structure in the subcortex, plays a major role in the psychological response to mental stress. Among its most common functions are temperature and hunger control; it also serves as the pleasure center. But, more important to this discussion, it is the area of the brain that governs the action of the *pituitary gland*, the body's master gland in charge of hormonal activity. The close interplay between the hypothalamus and the pituitary gland forms one of the major links between the mind and the body. Consider the following example of the way in which it works.

A negative event occurs in life, say a crash in the stock market. Through activities of the cortex, like reading and watching television news broadcasts, the event comes to the attention of the conscious mind, which immediately records the information and uses it to tell the individual that he has just lost a fortune because he had money invested. This entire process is simply a recognition and a deduction from the facts presented. It could have been performed by a computer, because it is purely rational, not emotional.

But through the actions of the limbic system, the event takes on a human component; it is associated with specific feelings and emotions. While these emotions can range from agony to ecstasy, in the example just presented they would most likely be unhappiness and worry, possibly even depression and despair. These emotions are then passed from the limbic system to the hypothalamus, which is suddenly alerted that something is wrong.

Once stimulated, the hypothalamus is compelled to relay these negative feelings to other areas of the brain. Since there is a strong connection between the hypothalamus and the pituitary gland, the gland gets jolted by strong and continuous input, messages that say, "The mind is in torment, prepare the body for some hard times." The pituitary responds accordingly by promoting the release of numerous hormones needed to maintain the individual through the crisis. While these hormones are essential to our well-being, in excessive amounts they cause serious internal damage—the physical result of prolonged mental stress.

Another connection between the brain and the body is the involuntary nervous system, also known as the *autonomic nervous system*. Unlike its partner, the voluntary nervous system, which controls conscious actions like walking or running, the autonomic system controls involuntary actions such as the secretion of fluids into the stomach or the constriction of blood vessels throughout the body. In response to mental stress, the autonomic nervous system triggers a well-known reaction called the "fight or flight" phenomenon, a common survival response noted throughout the animal kingdom.

The typical response goes something like this: When an animal is faced with a life-threatening situation, it must stand and fight or attempt to run away, thus the name "fight or flight." The physiological reaction that initiated the fight-or-flight response begins in the brain with the recognition of a perilous condition that must be immediately addressed. Accordingly, the autonomic nervous system unleashes a burst of activity that results in a massive release of adrenaline and the intense effects that this chemical has on the body. No doubt, you have witnessed this reaction in a common house cat that is unexpectedly confronted by a dog. Startled, the cat hunches its back, the hair on its neck rises, and the animal trembles and hisses. If you were observing the animal in a laboratory, you would see that its blood pressure rises and its heart races in response to blood shifting from the surface of its body into its brain and deep organs. If the cat were in the backyard, you would probably see it run to the nearest tree. But be assured, if cornered or unable to escape, the cat would be ready to fight for its life, aroused to super strength and cunning by the chemicals that flow through its body.

Occasionally the same reaction can be witnessed in human beings. For example, a woman lifts a car enough to free her husband who is trapped underneath, or a man plunges into freezing water to save someone who is drowning. In both cases, the superhuman response comes from the massive release of adrenaline that is part of the fight-or-flight phenomenon. However, unlike animals, which can fight or flee in response to a threatening event, people cannot always react aggressively. (Rarely does the man who loses a fortune in the stock market attack and kill his broker, although this can occur.) Instead, we usually control our emotions and maintain our composure—all at the expense of our health. When this happens, the chemicals of survival, the adrenaline and noradrenaline, transform into the chemicals of destruction, sacrificing rather than saving the individual. "Fight or flight" turns into acute stress, which works adversely in the body.

But how can this cause cancer? The answer begins with the pituitary gland, the master of the endocrine system, controlling all other hormone-producing organs in the body. It is located on the underside of the brain and communicates with the rest of the body through nerve connections and the blood. From its strategic location it monitors the rest of the endocrine glands and interacts closely with them.

Of the many endocrine glands, the adrenals play the most signficant role in the response to stress. During the response to mental stress, the hormones of the adrenal glands, *adrenaline* and *corticosteroids*, are released in abundance. The adrenaline quickly distributes to all parts of the body and, with the action of the hypothalamus, promotes the secretion of pituitary hormones. During short periods of stress, these adrenal and pituitary hormones perform many valuable functions that are essential to life itself. Yet over a period of days, weeks, or months, an excess secretion begins to take its toll. The stimulation of the adrenaline and of the thyroxin that flows from the thyroid cause a stressed individual to become irritable and restless. Sleep is often difficult, and physical exhaustion ensues. Over a prolonged period of time, the body is weakened, and the will to fight back diminishes. These feelings lead to more psychological distress, which only compounds the original emotional trauma. A vicious cycle is created and, if left unresolved, can physically and mentally destroy the individual.

Although this cycle has many components, of greatest interest to us in this discussion is the suppression of the immune system that occurs in the presence of *cortisol,* one of several corticosteroid hormones. The many functions of the corticosteroids include reducing the initial inflammatory response to injury and disease. The functions of the immune system also include recognizing foreign substances that enter or are produced in the body. Herein lies the connection between mental stress and cancer.

Because cancer cells are unnatural objects, members of the immune system recognize them as foreign invaders and immediately attack and destroy them before they can do damage. But what happens when the immune system is too incapacitated to identify early malignant cells or too weak to attack and destroy them? The following hospital case will dramatically illustrate the answer.

In the book *The Body Is Hero*, Ronald Glasser tells of a patient who underwent a normal kidney transplant but experienced a catastrophic setback a few days after surgery. Although the donor kidney had been well examined before it was transplanted, it apparently contained microscopic nodules of cancer that went undetected. As the patient was recuperating in the hospital, he started to go through some of the symptoms of rejection. The kidney began to enlarge rapidly, but continued to function—a very unusual pattern. To uncover the cause of this problem, a complete series of x-rays was taken, and to the amazement of everyone working on the case, tumors were found in the lungs. Since the lungs were completely clear before surgery, something must have occurred after the operation.

A second operation was quickly performed in order to examine the enlarged kidney. The surgeons found a huge fulminating malignancy. Clearly it was the source of the cancer that had spread to the lungs, but how could the growth have occurred so fast? After all, the kidneys and the lungs had appeared normal before the transplantation. The only possible cause: immunosuppressive drugs.

During all forms of transplant surgery, the patient receives numerous drugs to coerce the body to accept the donor organ. Since the donor organ is foreign—not of the same tissue type as the recipient's own organ—the cells of the immune system want to attack and destroy it, just as they would any invading virus, bacteria, or newly transformed cancer cell. But the action of the immunosuppressive drug prevents the immune system from acting normally, rendering it totally ineffective. Consequently, it cannot reject the kidney, but neither can it identify cancer cells. In the case just presented, the rapid growth of a microscopic tumor of the kidney into a massive spreading cancer well illustrates the consequence of a depressed immune system. It appropriately magnifies the problems that can be caused by the excessive secretion of cortisol, an immunosuppressive drug, from the adrenal glands in response to mentally generated stress.

Now what do you think happened to the cancerous kidney and the lung tumors when the immunosuppressive drugs were withdrawn from the patient's list of medication? The metastatic cancer in the lungs simply disappeared, and the cancer in the kidney retracted! The kidney eventually returned to normal size and was ultimately rejected. Left to an unfettered immune system, the cancer didn't have a chance. Of course, the patient had to be placed back on dialysis until a new kidney could be found, but at least he was free of cancer once again—brought back from a critical situation by his own natural defenses and the strength of his immune system!

That cortisol has the same effect on the immune system as immunosuppressive drugs is common knowledge within the medical community. In fact, corticosteroids like cortisol have been used therapeutically for years to reduce inflammation and temporarily reduce natural immunity. But the idea that the chronic release of cortisol in response to stress can lead to serious diseases like cancer is relatively recent news. Only over the past ten years has the direct connection between stress, cortisol release, and the development of malignancy been definitely established.

Cortisol: The Stress Hormone That Can Cause Cancer

In 1984 an article entitled "Stress, Cortisol, Interferon and 'Stress' Diseases" by Alfred T. Sapse appeared in *Medical Hypotheses*, a medical research journal. The evidence presented in the article showed that the elevated levels of cortisol chronically manufactured under the effect of prolonged stress are a primary cause of chronic illnesses, especially cancer. The information documenting cortisol's role in suppressing the immune system is plentiful:

- Cortisol reduces white blood cells (immune cells) in the thymus gland and in the lymph glands.

- It adversely affects specific groups of lymphocytes—T lymphocytes and T helpers.

- It increases the number of T supressor cells that limit the immune response.

- It inhibits the development of natural killer cells.

- It inhibits the growth of fibroblasts (fibrous tissue cells).

Since interferon, the antiviral, anticancer substance, is produced by T lymphocytes and fibroblasts, reduction in the number of these cells indirectly reduces the amount of interferon in the body, and consequently the ability to fight off viral disease and cancer.

In another report published in *Medical Hypotheses*, A. Klein showed that lymphocytes, in order to preserve their function and existence, actually can metabolize small amounts of cortisol. However, when cortisol levels are extreme, the lymphocyte's ability to survive is overwhelmed, and lymphocyte populations are diminished. Dr. Klein pointed out that these changes predate the growth of cancer.

Thus it is clear that cortisol levels in the body are crucial to overall welfare. Minute amounts are needed to assure good health and normal metabolic function, but excessive amounts are detrimental, reducing the number of immune cells and also their ability to properly perform in the face of adversity. The body must constantly maintain a delicate balance in order to preserve personal well-being. Without perceivable stress, this balance can be easily achieved.

One unusual group that demonstrates the connection between stress and cancer (or actually no stress and no cancer) is the collection of people classified as mentally handicapped. For quite some time, experts have noted that this group has a very low incidence of cancer.

Somehow, retarded individuals have a natural adversity to malignancy, with cancer rates far below the national average—14 percent compared to 17 percent in the general population. Initially it was thought that perhaps they had an unsually potent immune system that protected them from the threat of malignancy, but this theory has fallen from favor, since they regularly suffer from all the common infectious diseases of childhood and adult life, indicating that their natural defenses are no different than yours or mine. What then could explain their resistance?

With the establishment of the association between stress and cancer, another theory developed. If the mentally retarded have a limited understanding of life's events, they are less likely to experience the emotional turmoil that stems from stressful occurences. In turn, the messages that are sent from the mind to the body in normal individuals, the messages of sadness and sorrow, helplessness and hopelessness, are not generated in the mentally handicapped, and the entire process of cortisol release and the suppression of the immune system does not occur. Under these conditions, the immune cells of the retarded function normally and are highly successful in identifying and eliminating malignant cells before they have a chance to grow into an uncontrollable tumor. There is really nothing special about the natural defense systems of the mentally handicapped except that they are allowed to perform without restraint, without the limitations placed upon them by a keen conscious mind that translates unfortunate life happenings into emotional upheaval and a stressful bodily reaction.

Of course, severe stress cannot always be avoided; we all face it at different times in our lives. How we handle the stress and react to critical life events will determine how healthy we are and how well we handle the varied processes that cause malignant disease. We all have the natural tools and normal physiological functions to maintain strong, disease-free bodies, but we must use those tools properly and make our minds work in our favor. To do so, we must make certain changes in our lives, changes in the way we relate to our environment and in the way we respond to difficult circumstances. We must be able to identify the circumstances that generate overwhelming stress and to adjust ourselves accordingly. In essence, we must alter our personalities and psychological attitudes enough to cope with life's problems and influence the course of disease.

Psychological Factors

To support the theory that there are, indeed, personality traits and psychological states that can influence the way we handle malignancies, researchers have conducted thousands of studies into the subject, beginning as early as the eighteenth century. The collective results have shown that psychological and personality factors affect the body in innumerable ways and that the effect of life events significantly alters the state of mental and physical health, leaving the individual highly susceptible or making him completely immune to all forms of disease, including cancer. Simply put, the results suggest that each of us has the innate ability to generate illness or health; we have the power to control our own well-being.

In a review of emotional factors that contribute to malignant disease, Lawrence LeShan of the Institute of Applied Biology in New York summarized the idea that mental processes exert tremendous influence over our health. He reached several conclusions:

- Life events play major roles in establishing certain emotional and psychological states of mind.

- Specific psychological and emotional states are associated with the development and perpetuation of malignancy.

- The most common life event that creates the psychological and emotional condition that supports the growth of cancer is the loss of a close relationship.

- The strength of the personality determines the length of time that passes between the traumatic life event and the first-noted symptoms of cancer.

- The personality seems to be associated with the type or site of the cancer.

Without explanation, it is easy to see how life events, be they happy or sad, can affect our mental attitudes. Obviously, joyous events bring happiness and a beneficial mental disposition, while traumatic events generate anxiety, grief, depression, and the like. For quite some time, researchers have tried to measure the emotional effects of major life occurrences in order to make the associations more understandable and scientific. They have found that major events can be quantified in terms of the emotional stress they produce, and researchers have even designed a scale that numerically expresses these measurements. As you can see from the accompanying stress scale developed by Drs. T.H. Holmes and R.H. Rahe and adapted here, death of a spouse carries the most weight and has the single highest numerical value, indicating that it is the most traumatic event that can happen in a person's life. Next is divorce, then marital separation, and so on. Personal injury, change in financial status, family problems, and sexual difficulties all come into play and are assigned a numerical value that correlates to the degree of stress each of these events produces. The amount of emotional distress experienced by the individual relates to the stress factor and is associated with an initial outward manifestation that might include grief, remorse, anxiety, depression, or other negative psychological states. Even "positive" events, like Christmas, can cause stress.

SOCIAL READJUSTMENT RATING SCALE

EVENT	VALUE
Death of spouse	100
Divorce	73
Marital separation	65
Jail term	63
Death of close family member	63
Personal injury or illness	53
Marriage	50
Fired from work	47
Marital reconciliation	45
Retirement	45
Change in family member's health	44
Pregnancy	40
Sexual difficulties	39
Addition to family	39
Business readjustment	39
Change in financial status	38
Death of close friend	37
Change to different line of work	36
Change in number of marital arguments	36
Mortgage or loan over $10,000	31
Foreclosure of mortgage or loan	30
Change in work responsibilities	29
Son or daughter leaving home	29
Outstanding personal achievement	28
Spouse begins or stops work	26
Starting or finishing school	26
Change in living conditions	25
Revision of personal habits	24
Trouble with boss	23
Change in work hours, conditions	20
Change in residence	20
Change in schools	20
Change in recreational habits	19
Change in church activities	19
Change in social activities	18
Mortgage or loan under $10,000	17
Change in sleeping habits	16
Change in number of family gatherings	15
Change in eating habits	15
Vacation	13
Christmas season	12
Minor violation of the law	11

"The Social Readjustment Rating Scale" by T. H. Holmes and R. H. Rahe, *The Journal of Psychosomatic Research*, 1983, vol. II, pp. 213–218. Used with permission of the publisher, Pergamon Press, Inc.

Ancient scientists observed and recorded the emotional changes that accompany traumatic life occurrences. Studies from as early as the nineteenth century revealed a direct association between mental attitude and the growth of cancers. In 1846, Walter Hoyle Walshe commented extensively on the subject in a report, "The Nature and Treatment of Cancer," which became the definitive work of the time and clearly established the role of life's tragedies in creating psychological stress and a predisposition to cancer. Walshe cited mental misery, sudden reversals of fortune, and habitual gloominess as the most powerful forces that predispose an individual to cancer and said that these forces work through the mind to generate disease.

Today medical practitioners and researchers constantly make the same observations. In fact, using his stress scale, Dr. Holmes has been able to predict patients' statistical probabilities of developing cancer based on their psychological histories. He adds the values associated with the stress-related incidents in the previous twelve months of an individual's life. According to Holmes's findings, individuals who scored above 300 realized a 50 percent chance of contracting a serious illness, perhaps cancer. Additionally, individuals whose point scores were in the upper third of all patients studied reported 90 percent more illness than those who scored in the lower third of the entire group.

But not everyone who experiences several stressful events in a short period of time develops a serious illness. The statistics merely indicate an extreme predisposition based on psychological states of mind. Susceptibility appears to be affected by the strength of the individual's resolve and coping ability. This also seems to determine the length of time that passes between a tragic life happening and the initial indication of serious illness, as well as the speed at which the disease progresses or resolves.

The personality traits that make a person more susceptible to cancer develop from childhood, often stemming from the insecurity of a broken home, separation from one or both parents, and a lack of closeness to the father, mother, or both parents. Caroline Thomas of the Johns Hopkins University Department of Psychology identified lack of closeness with parents as a strong component in the psychological profiles of medical students who attended the Johns Hopkins School of Medicine and subsequently developed cancer later in life.

Likewise, Charles Goldfarb and his associates at St. Vincent's Medical Center in New York have identified several characteristics that are common to individuals stricken by cancer. As described in *Mind as Healer, Mind as Slayer* by Kenneth Pelletier, these include the inability to accept loss, immature sexual attitudes, difficulty in expressing hostility, maternal predominance, and feelings of hopelessness and helplessness. This sense of despondency was also observed by Drs. Schmale and Iker under similar circumstances. They conducted extensive psychological evaluations of their female patients and were able to predict, with a 73.6 percent degree of accuracy, which women would eventually develop malignancies and which would not.

Using psychological methods and in-depth interviews, it is not only possible to predict the likelihood of a malignant illness, it is also feasible to determine the most probable site of the malignancy. Problems with sexual attitudes (one component of the cancer profile), when associated with other cancer traits, frequently lead to cancer of the cervix or breast. This relationship was explored by two researchers, J.H. Stephenson and W.J. Grace, in a study entitled "Life Stress and Cancer of the Cervix," published in a medical journal called *Psychosomatic Medicine.* Stephenson and Grace reported that one of the oustanding sexual traits of the women interviewed was an extreme dislike of sexual intercourse. Other possible signs of poor sexual adjustment included failure to achieve orgasm, sexual infidelity, unfaithful husbands, separation, and a high incidence of divorce. All of these conditions occurred more frequently in women who developed cancer of the cervix than in women who developed cancers at other sites.

Another correlation exists between breast cancer and the psyche. For many years, it has been established that childless women who never had the opportunity to breast-feed were in some way predisposed to develop cancer of the breast. So too, were women who gave birth but didn't breast-feed. Initially, reserach pathologists assumed that the cancer arose because the breasts had not been able to perform their natural function of producing milk. Thus, through biological frustration, they were in some way disposed to develop cancer. However, Harold Voth, a psychiatrist at the Menninger Foundation, is reported in *Mind as Healer, Mind as Slayer* to feel that a more likely explanation is that disturbing childhood experiences generated a mental attitude that made nursing unacceptable or undesirable and thus predisposed the breast to psychologically encouraged illness. Of course, many other factors contribute to the development of breast cancer, but it is interesting that at least one cause has its source in the mind and emotions.

Likewise, lung cancer in men is associated with certain personal traits and a specific emotional profile. These factors were researched by David M. Kissen in a population of 366 male patients from three general hospitals. His findings show that the patients with lung cancer generally experienced childhood trauma arising from parental conflicts, which might have included separation or divorce. During their adult lives, these patients encountered serious problems at work or at home. Interpersonal relationships were problematic, and the men typically had difficulty venting their emotions. Also significant was the duration of the adult problems. Difficulties were unusually long-standing and contributed to mental stress for inordinate lengths of time, frequently longer than ten years.

While these studies were set up to look into the histories of cancer patients in order to shed light on psychological factors that relate to the evolution of malignant disease, they also provide a way of looking into the future in order to predict potential physical problems. As Pelletier points out in his wonderful book, "Research concerning these types of cancers suggests that, by analyzing the personality and the emotional characteristics which precede them, it may be possible to look at other individuals and to predict the site at which a future cancer will develop." More importantly, with an understanding of the connection between the mind and the body, between personality traits and the reaction to life events, it becomes possible to make the adjustments necessary to prevent cancer from developing or continuing to grow. By learning to control the forces of the mind, you can reduce stress and shut down the excessive flow of cortisol that weakens the immune system and fosters or sustains growth of malignant cells. In effect, you can turn off the BAD SYSTEM and turn on the GOOD SYSTEM.

TURNING ON THE GOOD SYSTEM

By balancing mental and physical forces, achieving a true harmony between the mind and the body, you will turn on the GOOD SYSTEM, the anticancer system. The GOOD SYSTEM will not provide the environment in which cancer can grow, nor the harmful substances that stimulate malignant growth, nor the stifling of the immune system that allows the growth to continue. On the contrary, the GOOD SYSTEM, associated with positive mental attitudes and a strong, healthy body, is the system that operates under the influence of the substances of good health, the miracle chemicals—the endorphins and enkephalins that flow from the brain and the interferon and interleukin that are produced by the body. It is the system with a potent natural defense composed of white blood cells that stand ready to fight the malignant enemy. It is the system of wholeness and life.

Each of these systems can exist within you. Your own desire and determination will decide which one it will be—the GOOD or the BAD. If you now have cancer, you have probably been functioning under the influence of the BAD SYSTEM for some time. Perhaps excess daily stress has brought about the illness in your body, or maybe it was a poor mental attitude combined with harmful personality traits, or possibly poor eating habits and a lack of daily exercise.

Regardless, it's time to make a change for the better, to reassert control and turn the tide on cancer. By adjusting yourself properly, you can eliminate the conditions that support and maintain cancer. By altering your mental state, you can cause the release of all the wonderful chemicals of the GOOD SYSTEM, the chemicals of faith, hope, and love. To achieve your goal of total cancer elimination and a complete and lasting cure, to turn off the BAD SYSTEM and turn on the GOOD SYSTEM, you must push the right buttons.

The Amazing Story of Norman Cousins

Perhaps the most amazing example of turning off the BAD SYSTEM and turning on the GOOD SYSTEM is the wonderful story of Norman Cousins. It dramatically demonstrates the power of laughter in changing mental attitude and competely reversing a life-threatening physical condition. Like a powerful drug—a natural cure-all—good humor restored Mr. Cousins to good health as he literally laughed his way out of the hospital. Since his story was so unusual at the time (1964) and so revealing in its scope, it was widely discussed within medical communities around the world and eventually published as a reflection on healing and regeneration in *Anatomy of an Illness as Perceived by the Patient*, written by Mr. Cousins himself, an excellent writer and a longtime editor with the *Saturday Review*.

"I have learned," writes Mr. Cousins, "never to underestimate the capacity of the human mind and body to regenerate—even when the prospects seem most unfavorable. The life-force may be the least understood force on earth." He came to this realization after personally directing and simultaneously witnessing his miraculous recovery from illness. Norman Cousins went from a hospitalized patient given one chance in 500 of living to a man well enough to write and lecture about his experience. Truly his story is a shining example of our ability to cure ourselves.

Mr. Cousins's illness began in August 1964 with fever and fatigue that quickly led to stiffness in his neck, arms, legs, hands, and fingers. In the days that followed the onset of symptoms, his condition worsened until he was confined to a hospital bed, unable to move. His own description of the experience is chilling. "I had considerable difficulty in moving my limbs and even turning over in bed. Nodules appeared on my body, gravel-like substances under the skin, indicating the systemic nature of the disease. At the low point of my illness, my jaws were almost locked shut."

After too many tests to mention here, he was finally given the horrible news from a full staff of doctors working on his case. Apparently he suffered from a terminal collagen disease and had but one chance in 500 of ever recovering. Incredibly, miraculously, and to the astonishment of medical experts, he managed to beat the odds.

Defying medical authorities and gambling heavily on the outcome, he transferred himself out of the hospital into a hotel and took himself off medication. He initiated his self-treatment by taking large doses of vitamin C and implementing a plan to improve his mental attitude. If negative emotions had a negative effect on the body, as he was inclined to believe after reading *The Stress of Life* by Hans Selye, then, he reasoned, positive emotions must have a positive effect. On this belief he based his therapy.

Each day, his nurse was instructed to play funny movies for him and to read from humorous books—anything to provoke laughter. From the very onset, Cousins noticed that ten minutes of hearty laughter would leave him pain-free for at least two hours and allow him to sleep. The sleep itself undoubtedly aided in his recovery, which was monitored by the same lab tests that had previously exposed the severity of his condition. The combination of vitamin C and laughter seemed to be working.

"At the end of the eighth day I was able to move my thumbs without pain. By this time, the elevated sedimentation rate (one of the many lab tests used to monitor the course of the illness) was somewhere in the 80's and was resolving quickly. I couldn't be sure, but it seemed to me that the gravel-like nodules on my neck and back of my hands were beginning to shrink. There was no doubt in my mind that I was going to make it back all the way."

While Mr. Cousins's health steadily improved, the process was slow. For months he could not raise his arms completely or fully turn his head. He was forced to wear knee braces in order to walk and suffered from pain for well over a year. But the suffering and the pain eventually disappeared, and the results were overwhelmingly positive. Norman Cousins made a full recovery. He went full circle from death's grip to life's sweet embrace, using the natural ability of his mind and body to fight his illness and produce a spontaneous remission. In Norman Cousins's case, treating his illness meant tickling his funny bone.

Mr. Cousins's mental attitude had a distinctly positive role in the recovery from his illness. What he had discovered was that the mind has the potential to positively affect the body during periods of joy and happiness, hope and faith. He had tapped into the chemicals of good health and positive emotions.

These recently discovered substances, called *neurochemicals*, account for the health benefits of happiness and contentment. Neurochemicals serve as the link between positive thinking and physical well-being, and they unlock the mysteries of the mind-body connections. As they pertain to curing cancer, the neurochemicals of the GOOD SYSTEM are potentially the most important substances in cancer research today, since they literally hold the key to the future, not only for scientists and doctors, but for all those of us who wish to influence our own longevity.

Natural Uppers

From his research in the late 1970s, Carl Simonton developed the concept that conscious effort on the part of the patient can turn the course of cancer in the patient's favor. He viewed the process as a reversal of the cycle that produced the malignancy in the first place and explained the phenomenon in this way.

First, there is psychological reinforcement of the effectiveness of treatment. The patient truly believes that he or she has been helped by the doctors, family members and friends. The patient comes to believe in the power of his or her own natural defense system and its ability to continue the fight against the disease. The patient also develops the faith that he or she will be cured.

Next there is an improvement in the patient's overall outlook on life. The problems that were so troubling before the onset of the disease now appear in a different light. Once viewed as unsolvable and inescapable, they are now seen as circumstances that can be controlled. With this new outlook on life and the belief that therapy and personal support will overcome the illness, the patient's vision of the future contains hope.

The hope and positive outlook are recorded by the limbic system and replace the previous feelings of helplessness and hopelessness. Messages that reflect these new feelings are sent to the hypothalamus, which in turn sends to the pituitary gland the news that the patient's emotional status has changed.

The pituitary gland then takes over. Previously, during the period of stress and negative feelings, the pituitary had been pumping out chemicals that affected the adrenals, thyroid, and other endocrine glands. In response, these glands released their individual hormones, which became the chemicals of destruction—the ingredients of the BAD SYSTEM that contribute to the creation and sustenance of cancer. But with a more positive psychological state in operation and the conveyance of hope from the conscious mind to the physical body, the pituitary gland's excessive stimulation of the entire endocrine system is halted, and a natural balance of hormones is reestablished.

Now, instead of disrupting and suppressing the immune system, the chemicals of positive emotions actually stimulate the natural defense system to rally a response against the cancer. New cancer cells do not arise, and existent cells are destroyed through the actions of the white blood cells and the anticancer chemicals of a strong and healthy immune complex. Slowly but surely, the cancer is brought under control until it is virtually eliminated and the patient goes into total remission.

The positive effects of a healthy mental attitude are broadly demonstrated in real life by numerous and diverse groups. As examples, consider the Unity and New Thought congregations. Within these sects, religious teachings include the necessity of living in harmony with all things, of maintaining an excellent level of health, and of visualizing one's self as an intricate part of God's perfection. Religious teachings include the practice of healing with the imagination and of achieving a state of perfect health through the powers of the mind and will. These groups suffer far less frequently from the common ailments that plague today's societies and seem to recover much more rapidly if illness does strike. They also record far fewer sick days than the general work force and have a lower incidence of cancer than the national average. Undoubtedly, it is the positive image they hold of themselves that protects them from illnesses and greatly assists them in their recoveries.

The centenarian societies practice a similar sort of visualization, only more subtly. Within the older populations, the view of one's self contains a vision of a long and healthy life. Individuals expect to live beyond their 100th birthday, and they do. They view themselves as productive members of society for as long as they live, and consequently they do function effectively even in their eighties, nineties, and one-hundreds. Their positive vision of themselves keeps them going. It is the self-fulfilling prophecy of their own minds.

Other important qualities of life also appear to encourage well-being and longevity, plus a low occurrence of malignant disease. Family support and personal security seem to play a significant role in the maintenance of good health, as demonstrated by the daily lives of the Seventh Day Adventists. Members of this group share a common code of mutual assistance and cooperative support, not only spiritually and emotionally, but also financially. Any member of the group who needs something can obtain it within the group from people who care about each other and are willing to help in any way possible. This support creates strong personal security and a feeling of being loved and cared for at all times and in all situations. Can you imagine the positive benefits to your health that these kinds of feelings can bestow? Statistically these benefits have been shown to be real, including a lower than usual incidence of cancer.

The initial discovery of the chemicals of euphoria occurred in the late 1960s and early 1970s when scientists found that stimulating the brain with minute electrical shocks could alleviate physical pain and create a feeling of well-being. The next discovery revealed that numerous areas throughout the brain contain natural receptors for narcotic-like substances, opiates, that produce an analgesia similar to that from heroin or morphine. Finally, several doctors independently discovered a group of naturally occurring substances that would bind to these receptor sites and also produce some of the pain-killing effects first noted with the electrical stimulation. These new chemicals were called endorphins, a name that refers to the type of substances they are— endogenous opioid peptides, or simply opium-like proteins.

The endorphins are manufactured by nerve tissue in specific areas in the brain. Some of those locations, like the limbic system, mentioned earlier in this chapter, are directly associated with the link between the mind and the body. Additional sites of endorphin production are in the thalamus and the brain's deep internal gray matter, plus the areas that are affiliated with mood and control of the endocrine system. Their location alone indicates that these substances are intimately connected with the mind-body response.

Perhaps the most publicized effect of the endorphins is their ability to eliminate pain. Their release during childbirth is a well-documented fact, and it is the endorphins' action that greatly reduces the overall pain a mother feels when she gives birth. Without the presence of the endorphins, natural childbirth might be all but impossible because of the intense pain associated with the event.

During athletic events such as long-distance running, the endorphins keep the competitors going. Endorphins are said to help marathon runners make it through "the wall," the toughest section of a race, the stretch around 18 miles when the body wants to give out but the mind draws all the strength it can muster and bursts with endorphins to push the runner to his or her highest effort.

These magical substances are also associated with heroic achievements, when individuals overcome tremendous opposition in meeting insurmountable challenge or conquering a formidable foe. So too, are they released during periods of great pain, when a person, by all rights, should be incapacitated. Obviously, they are of immense importance to our emotional and physical well-being and to our very survival.

Unlike their direct effects on the pain of childbirth or the endurance of long-distance runners, endorphins have an indirect effect on cancer. As part of the GOOD SYSTEM, they are like a powerful drug prescribed from the pharmacy of the mind, and when present in sufficient quantity, their actions greatly assist the body's natural defense system to fight its never-ending battle against the malignant threat.

Recent scientific evidence indicates that endorphins enhance the power of the immune system in fighting disease in general and cancer in particular. In 1982, at the Second International Conference on Immunopharmacology (the study of substances that effect the immune system), N.P. Plotnikoff presented a report (described in Jeanne Achterberg's *Imagery in Healing*) that documented the increased potential of T lymphocytes in cancer patients who had elevated levels of endorphins in their blood. In addition, further study by other independent researchers has proven the existence of endorphin receptors on the surface of lymphocytes, thereby indicating that the chemical probably has a direct stimulating effect on the immune cell. Beta-endorphins have been shown to increase the ability of T lymphocytes to proliferate so that their numbers can increase in response to a malignant challenge. Another type of endorphin, called enkephalin, increases the number of active T lymphcytes that aggressively seek out and destroy cancer cells. Clearly, all of these effects are of great benefit to the cancer patient, who requires the strongest immune system possible and an expanded number of highly aggressive immune cells. Endorphins seem to aid in both respects.

Another aid to the immune system is the naturally occurring substance histamine, which is intimately connected with emotions. As part of the inflammation response of allergies, histamine has shown its potent effect on blood flow and immune cells. Since it is associated with feelings and immediate psychological responses to sexual activity, it might be mentally controllable, which brings us to the final point of this chapter. Can an individual directly, through conscious effort, control the release of all these substances and perhaps others still to be identified? If so, how?

The Mind's Positive Power

According to Jeanne Achterberg, whose wonderful book, *Imagery in Healing*, is must reading for those who go on to practice visualization as part of their adjunct therapy, the brain and the immune system are consciously connected. There must be experiments that can verify changes in the immune response of individuals who manage to turn their mental attitudes around and replace hopelessness with hope and sadness with joy. After creating an intricate testing program and overcoming problems with blood samples and testing centers, she arrived at the following analysis.

Differences in blood chemistry and mental attitude divided patients into three groups. One group, in which patients had an attitude of resignation and a negative psychological disposition, was found to have severe blood deficiencies. Another group, characterized by worry, anxiety, and a directionless psychological struggle, had a deficiency of red blood cells, yet no significant alteration in white cells. The third group, classified as the fighters, demonstrated the desire to overcome their illness through direct and purposeful action, and showed a higher than normal white blood cell count. Achterberg and her associates interpreted this increase in white blood cells as a strengthening of the natural immune system, which heavily relies on both the T and B lymphocytes in the reaction that leads to remissions.

In Achterberg's own words, "The overriding conclusion was that, within the sample studied, there were three differing psychological profiles that appeared to represent a sort of continuum, starting from an attitude of giving up, extending to an attitude of ambivalent struggle, and finally reaching to include a purposeful and positive striving to overcome the disease. These were related to distinct blood profiles. Only in the most positive profile was the immune system seen to be enhanced." More simply put, the "fighters" who demonstrated a positive attitude and a purposeful response in dealing with their disease also had blood chemistries that indicated a stronger immune system. An increase in lymphocytes, the white blood cells that destroy cancer, was the single most important factor in the improved blood profile. The studies clearly demonstrated that attitude can indeed change blood chemistries for the better or for the worse, and it is the chemicals of hope, the endorphins and other similar substances, that cause the changes that increase our odds of survival.

We all manufacture these remarkable substances of the GOOD SYSTEM, and we all experience the benefits of these wonderful compounds day by day. More importantly, we have the power to purposefully cause their release and effectively use them to fight our illnesses. When controlled properly and adequately, the chemicals of the GOOD SYSTEM help rid the body of cancer and stimulate spontaneous remissions. It's up to us to bring all of these elements into play.

II
YOUR BODY
HEALER

7
Macrobiotics and the Remission of Cancer

Anthony Satillaro examined his own chest X-ray with understandable concern. As an experienced physician and thirteen-year chairman of the anesthesiology department at Methodist Hospital in Philadelphia, he knew all too well that the large mass in the left side of his chest indicated a serious problem, most likely a tumor. He also realized that immediate attention to the problem was absolutely essential, so he wisely submitted himself for some additional tests.

First on the list was a bone scan; preparation began at once with an intravenous injection of radioactive dye. A few hours later, after the dye had evenly spread throughout his system, Dr. Satillaro found himself flat on his back under a computerized scanner that would locate any abnormal skeletal accumulation of radioactive material. Watching the telltale monitor as the scanner passed over his body, he shuddered in disbelief at what he saw. First a mass of radioactivity appeared in his skull, another in his back. According to the scanner, Dr. Satillaro had widespread cancer. He revolted. "My skin was suddenly galvanized by a wave of adrenalin and body heat. I got up from the table and wanted to vomit," he recalled later.

Additional tests and tissue studies proved that Dr. Satillaro, forty-six years old, had prostatic cancer, grade 4D—a very unkind diagnosis that carries a short survival rate of eighteen-to-thirty-six months. Obviously, if he expected to reach his fiftieth birthday, he had no time to waste. So Dr. Satillaro became Patient Satillaro and began a personal drama that held his very life in the balance. At a whirlwind pace, surgery was performed, followed by hormone therapy, in an attempt to remove as much cancer as possible and to suppress the rest. But the postoperative period proved exceptionally difficult, and the months that followed found Satillaro constantly in pain, suffering numerous physical and personal setbacks, including the cancer death of his father. Despair is obvious in his own recollections: "My cancer did not seem to be controlled, my pain was worse than ever, and in attending my father's funeral, I almost felt as if I had attended my own."

Then, through an unlikely sequence of events, Satillaro's life changed. Returning home to Philadelphia from his father's funeral in Hopelawn, New Jersey, he picked up two outspoken hitchhikers who, in a manner of speaking, indirectly rerouted him to the East West Holistic Health Foundation and its director, Denny Waxman.

Like the two opinionated strangers before him, Waxman spouted the belief that both the cause and cure of cancer are related to diet. Therein, he claimed, resides the key to good health. Unbelieving, Dr. Satillaro listened. Although skeptical of dietary therapy, especially as a cure for cancer, Satillaro found himself desperately searching for help and hope, and he somehow viewed Waxman as a possible source of both. He was taken in and for seven months ate macrobiotic food at the table of Judy and Denny Waxman.

Brown rice, whole grains, vegetables, soybeans, seaweed, soup, and condiments—pure, wholesome and therapeutic—were the foundation of the diet. Meat, dairy products, oils, sugar, white flour, alcohol, and processed foods were taboo, poisons to be avoided. Satillaro was placed on the strictest diet possible, since his condition was critical. But could it have an effect? Was it worthwhile? These questions and hundreds more passed through his mind.

He relates, "I had real problems accepting Denny's argument. To suggest that diet was the root of cancer seemed like an incredible oversimplification of the etiology of this disease. Waxman's line of reasoning did not take into account several other possible causes of cancer, including genetic disposition, viruses, and carcinogens in the environment. Yet I knew I would continue to eat at the Waxmans'."

As time passed, Satillaro did more than just eat. Gradually he began to participate in discussions about macrobiotic foods, and slowly but steadily he gained a better understanding and appreciation of the macrobiotic diet. Eventually, like a curious schoolboy whose enthusiasm and interest grow with his level of understanding, Satillaro became preoccupied and pleasantly distracted by the diet and the macrobiotic philosophy. The more he learned, the more he wanted to know, until the diet became an intricate part of his daily life. But was it beneficial? September 26, 1978, brought the answer to that question.

When Satillaro awoke at 6:30 A.M. he instinctively reached for the bottle of painkillers that he had religiously taken every day. But that day was different; something had changed. It took Satillaro only a couple of minutes to realize that he didn't need the medication because his back pain was gone. After months of suffering, the pain had suddenly disappeared. In the weeks that followed, a variety of intestinal problems also cleared, and Satillaro's vitality and energy seemed to be substantially heightened. While these personal evaluations hinted at improvement, they were only subjective observations. The concrete evidence was yet to come.

In January, new lab tests showed a remarkable improvement—significantly greater than was expected from the treatments that Satillaro had received. A bone scan was subsequently scheduled.

As radioactive dye was again injected into his veins, Tony was advised not to be disappointed if the results were less than what he was hoping for. Bones, after all, take a long time to heal, and radical improvement should not be expected. With these thoughts in mind, he reclined under the scanner and observed the monitor as the machine passed over his body from head to toe.

Again, Satillaro was overcome by what he saw, only this time it was joy, not horror, that saturated his senses. No tumor in his skull. None in his shoulder, rib cage, or sternum. Nothing in his back. No cancer anywhere. Miraculously, he was rid of the horrible disease.

Follow-up studies have continued to give Satillaro a clean bill of health, except for a minor setback that was subsequently overcome. His doctors have proclaimed a "complete remission." Still, constant monitoring is necessary to pick up any possible recurrence.

Satillaro's case is rare but understandable. As was Norman Cousins, whose faith in the power of laughter and good humor restored him to good health, Anthony Satillaro was cured through his faith in adherence to the macrobiotic diet. Both men managed to push the buttons that turned off the BAD SYSTEM and turned on the GOOD. Both men saved their own lives by using the powers of their minds and bodies to generate their remission.

Another case that reflects the power of the macrobiotic diet took place in 1978 at the Vermont Medical Center. The patient, a middle-aged woman, was diagnosed as having stage 4 malignant melanoma of the skin—a rapidly growing cancer in an advanced state. Her doctor recommended the traditional treatment for this type of cancer: wide excisional biopsy with additional removal of the local lymph glands to catch any possible spread of malignant cells. He also commented that follow-up therapy based on the initial surgical findings might be necessary. Much to the doctor's surprise and chagrin, the patient refused his recommendations and treatment. Although she had training in the medical field, she had always advocated alternative therapies. Yet she knew she had failed to heed her own advice and had fallen victim to a poor diet, personal frustration, and stress. She viewed her cancer as a personal challenge and endeavored to cure it on her own.

On a recommendation from her son, she visited the East West Foundation Cancer Center in Amherst, Massachusetts, and started on a standard macrobiotic diet the same day. Impressed with the initial results, she attended advanced courses and learned more about the macrobiotic diet and lifestyle. She persevered with the program and received its rewards.

Within the first week of therapy, she noticed improvement. She regained much of her former energy and also improved her mental attitude and clarity. From the low point of her condition, when she could hardly make it up a flight of stairs, she progressed to exercising every day—a dramatic improvement in her eyes. She herself was amazed by her perseverance, and her determination undoubtedly assisted in her recovery, not only because she adhered faithfully to the diet but because she was stimulated to seek out more information and to become more emotionally involved. She rapidly progressed in the understanding and elimination of her health problems and brought herself to a point in October 1979 when she was pronounced "cured" of cancer. Wisely, she has continued to adhere to the macrobiotic way of life and to share her experience and knowledge with those who need her help. Although she took great risks in avoiding conventional therapy, risks that I wouldn't personally recommend, in her case everything worked out well.

A final case involves an ovarian illness. The patient's problems began in the spring of 1978, when she developed frequent and painful menstrual periods. Initially, her doctor had difficulty diagnosing the condition, but after examination and study, the doctor concluded that the patient had a dermoid tumor of the right ovary—a diagnosis that was also supported by a second physician. Since it was impossible to determine whether the tumor was benign or malignant, the doctors advised an immediate operation. The ovary and the tumor would be removed, then examined by a pathologist who would establish a definitive diagnosis. Regardless of the outcome, the patient was going to have to lose her ovary.

Before consenting to the surgery, this patient, like the one discussed previously, decided to take a great risk and try to heal herself through macrobiotics only, a therapy with which she was only vaguely familiar. She attended a seminar on the subject at Amherst College near Boston, where she learned about the diet and the benefit it had provided others. Applying this new knowledge to her own life, she returned home and began to make the necessary changes to overcome her illness.

From the beginning, she had faith in the power of macrobiotics, and she continued to believe that she could heal herself. The more she learned, the more she was convinced that conventional treatments would ultimately become unnecessary and that she would indeed overcome the disease on her own. As time went on, her thoughts became reality.

Slowly her symptoms began to subside; the back pain eased, and her periods reverted to normal. Upon returning to her original doctor for a reevaluation some six months after the first visits, she was relieved but not amazed to learn that the orange-sized tumor had disappeared. Her doctor could find no trace of it but was at a loss to explain how it had vanished. Four months later, during another checkup, the patient was informed that the ovary had returned to normal. Without any treatment other than the macrobiotic therapy, the patient was not only cured, but actually normal again.

In retrospect, the "miracle" was in large part due to the macrobiotic diet, but in the mind of the patient the support she had received from the East West Foundation in Boston was also invaluable. It had bolstered her faith and given her the strength to continue. As she put it, "My faith was as important as the diet itself. . . . The support I had received in following the macrobiotic diet and the way of life was also very important."

In the book entitled *Healing Miracles through Macrobiotics* by Gene Kohler et al, there are a variety of testimonials about cancer cures attributed solely to the macrobiotic diet. Like the three examples presented here, they provide vivid illustrations of the value of this type of therapy. To show how this therapy works, this chapter describes some of the basic principles of the macrobiotic philosophy.

PRINCIPLES AND THEORIES OF MACROBIOTICS

Cancer is a disease of many causes, or, more precisely, it is many diseases of many causes. For a number of years, experts have tried to establish a universal theory to explain its occurrence. From various specialties in medical science have come varied ways of interpreting the disease and numerous ways of treating it. From the macrobiotic point of view, all cancers are caused by the body's attempt to maintain a balance. A cancer grows in a particular area in order to *detoxify* the rest of the body. In other words, the cancer accumulates carcinogens in one location in order to allow the remaining organs to function normally. From what we know about the disease, except in the final stages of illness, a

body with a malignant tumor does indeed function
without noticeable change and generally gives no indication whatsoever that something is amiss. So, in a
sense, a delicate balance is maintained. According to
macrobiotic teaching, that balance can be considered,
temporarily, a means of self-protection.

But what causes the carcinogenesis? According to
macrobiotics, the answer is food.

For over three decades now, independent researchers
and agencies have conducted studies of the association
between food and disease. All over the world, data from
animal experiments and human studies have been collected linking certain diets with certain illnesses. Today, the link between diet and cancer is undeniable.

A quick review of the many animal studies turns up
numerous associations. For example, in 1961, two researchers, Drs. Wood and Larson, hunted for the cause
of an outbreak of liver cancer in cultured trout from an
Idaho hatchery. Through their investigations, they determined that the only possible explanation was a simple change in diet. Unprocessed meal had been fed to
the fish for years, contributing to healthy harvests.
With a switch to processed meal containing unnatural
ingredients came the unprecedented liver cancer. It
was an open-and-shut case.

Other animal studies have shown a direct correlation
between cancer and excess food consumption. Simply,
increased cancer deaths and decreased longevity have
been related to obesity in laboratory animals.

Human research supports the same vital conclusion:
Cancer is related to diet. For example, in 1963, a study
compared the rates of three different cancers, stomach,
breast, and colon, among Americans and Japanese. It
was shown that before 1947 the Japanese had a much
higher rate of stomach cancer, six times higher. The
Americans were more prone to breast and colon cancer,
two to three times more prone. Why? Before 1947, the
Japanese diet contained high quantities of white rice,

sugar, vinegar, monosodium glutamate, and artificial seasonings, while the American diet contained large amounts of animal foods like meat, milk, and cheese, along with sugar and soft drinks. Then, after 1947 and the postwar reconstruction of Japan, the Japanese diet was significantly westernized, and interesting changes began to occur.

As the Japanese consumption of milk increased twenty-three times and the egg consumption increased thirteen times, with meats and other "American" foods on the increase as well, the Japanese began to suffer "American" diseases. The occurrence of stomach cancer diminished 33 percent, but breast and colon cancer increased to approximately American levels. With a change in diet came a change in disease; similar diets produced similar illnesses.

More evidence to support this study was provided by Japanese immigrants to America. As they left their homelands and their native diets to relocate in a new land with novel foods, they also exchanged their typically Eastern illnesses for problems that were basically Western. After only three generations, the cancer rates for stomach and colon malignancies adjusted to the American standards.

There are other correlations as well. Within the United States, people who consume similar foods usually maintain a similar degree of health and suffer from similar illnesses. Vegetarian groups such as the Seventh Day Adventists, for example, have significantly lower cancer rates than their meat-eating counterparts. Likewise, individuals forced into vegetarian diets enjoy similar benefits. As a case in point, consider the following account.

During the German occupation of Holland in World War II, the standard diet underwent great modification. Since the Germans requisitioned much of the available meat, cheese, milk, butter, and eggs, the Dutch were forced to eat vegetables, grains, breads, and other basic foodstuffs. Interestingly, the incidence of cancer among the Dutch dropped by rates of 35 percent to 60 percent, depending on the geographic location. When conditions returned to normal after the war, higher cancer rates also returned.

Similar studies abound throughout the medical literature, and the relationship between diet and disease is well established. Over the past ten years, in fact, more than two dozen international health organizations have produced studies that cite diet as a major factor in the development of most diseases, and many of these organizations have made recommendations regarding the prevention of illness through a sensible daily diet.

Macrobiotic experts go one step further. They not only recognize the connection between certain foods and the development of cancer, they firmly believe that a change of diet will reverse the cancerous process and actually eliminate the disease, even when standard therapy is abandoned.

The principle behind the macrobiotic diet is the theory that all things in the universe are a balance of two opposing yet complementary forces—expansion and contraction. These forces create a balance or harmony that perpetuates all processes in nature. They are the powers that keep the universe expanding but also intact. They are the constantly changing components of energy and matter so simply expressed by Albert Einstein as $E = mc^2$. To use more familiar examples, these forces include such common pairs as the positive and negative polarity of a magnet, the north and south polarity of the Earth, the dual nature of the sexes as male and female, and the give and take of the life force within our bodies—the positive and negative elements that drive our physical beings.

In the field of macrobiotics, the two forces are called yin and yang, and all things can be classified as one or the other. Classifying foods as either yin or yang is an essential component of the macrobiotic philosophy and diet. The distinction lies in the growth characteristics and composition of the food. For example, foods grown in a hot climate are yin; those grown in a cold climate are yang. Fruits and leafy vegetables are yin, but stems, roots, and seeds are classified as yang. Sour, bitter, and sweet foods are also yin, while salty and pungent foods are yang. The classification becomes very specific, to the point that all foods are categorized as one type or the other. For instance, oranges are yin, and carrots are yang.

Likewise, the organs of the body are separated into the yin and yang classes. The hollow and expansive organs, like the stomach and the intestines, fall into the yin category, whereas the solid and condensed body parts, like the liver or pancreas, occupy the list of yang organs. Although the evaluation becomes more exacting and complex with the classification of specific parts of different organs, it is sufficient to know that each organ has a predominant characteristic of either yin or yang.

Finally we come to the cancers themselves. Be it breast cancer or cancer of the bone, brain cancer or cancer of the blood, every malignancy has its own classification, falling into one category or the other. This categorization is of great importance because it directs the individual in the proper choice of foods from the macrobiotic menu. When a cancer is predominantly yin, it is most appropriately treated by a diet that emphasizes yang foods. Yang cancers require treatment with predominantly yin diets. In either case, all extreme foods—those that are excessively yin or yang in nature—should be totally avoided. Adjusting the diet to accentuate foods that diametrically oppose the quality of the cancer creates a natural balance and reverses the forces that sustain the malignancy.

MACROBIOTIC TEACHINGS

In macrobiotic teaching, cancer is viewed as a disease of excess. Therefore, it is important for the cancer patient not to overeat and further contribute to the excessive condition. One neat principle of the diet that reduces the hunger and consequently the food intake, is the belief in chewing thoroughly. Each bite should be chewed at least fifty and preferably one hundred times. This completely pulverizes the food and thoroughly mixes it with saliva, which is rich in amylase, an enzyme that breaks down simple carbohydrates. Digestion literally starts in the mouth and enhances the digestive functions of the stomach, providing for more rapid absorption in the intestines. The benefit is twofold. First, as the food is absorbed, blood sugar rises and satiates the appetite. Second, since the food is chewed over and over again, consumption is delayed while hunger diminishes. Consequently, less food is desired, and less is eaten.

Another important recommendation is the caution not to eat at least three hours before retiring for the night. The body does not properly use food eaten just before going to sleep. It will be deposited as fat or other undesirable substances and enhance the development of malignancies.

In the basic diet, grains, beans, and vegetables predominate. These should be mixed to ensure the ingestion of all the amino acids that are essential for complete protein synthesis and should be adjusted to emphasize an opposing balance to the nature of the cancer. The consumption of fatty animal foods is strictly prohibited. These include red meat, poultry, dairy items, eggs, and all other oily or greasy items. Fish may be eaten once or twice a week by individuals with yin cancers but should be avoided completely by patients with yang disorders. Nuts and seeds may be consumed infrequently and only when the problem is yang in nature. Since fruits are extremely yin, they are not recommended but may occasionally be eaten by individuals with yang illnesses.

As mentioned, vegetables constitute a large part of

the macrobiotic diet. Since they are neither excessively yin nor overly yang, they may be consumed by patients with both forms of cancer. The major consideration in their use is preparation. In cases of yin cancers, vegetables should be cooked slowly and thoroughly with an emphasis on boiling. Tamari or miso seasoning may be used. For yang cancers, boiling should be rapid and short so that the vegetables are still crisp and fresh. Sautéing them quickly on a high flame is also allowed, and they may be modestly seasoned with sea salt.

The only recommended beverages are water and green and bancha stem teas. The teas come from different parts of the same bush and are harvested at different times. The green tea tends to be more yin, and the bancha stem tea is more yang. The highest recommendation goes to the bancha stem tea, also known as kukicha. Made from the stems and branches of the plant, it is an excellent beverage for all cancer patients and may be consumed as much as desired. Processed or aromatic teas are to be avoided altogether.

Much more specific advice about what to eat and how to prepare it is available from reliable and concerned sources throughout the United States and the rest of the world. Presented here is just an overview of the macrobiotic diet that provides a glimpse into its nature and philosophy. As a cancer-fighting weapon, it is powerful. Not only does it balance the dietary forces of yin and yang to reverse previous toxicities, it also promotes significant alterations in the body's chemistry, creating an unsuitable environment for cancer.

At the commencement of the diet, the patient will find it difficult to maintain such a rigid regimen of eating habits. After the first day, the patient will doubt that he or she can tolerate the diet. But after a few days, the positive effects begin to shine through. First of all, the person begins to feel better. The sluggish, sedentary feelings produced by overeating will dissipate, and the individual will be more energetic and animated.

Next, an innovative and motivating strength will arise with the patient's realization that he or she has taken a decisive step and already feels some benefits. This feeling will grow, and soon the patient will believe that he or she can turn the illness around through personal intervention. The mind becomes stronger along with the body, and the cancer becomes weaker as the chemicals of the GOOD SYSTEM are released in abundance. Endorphins begin to flow from the brain, and the immune system is greatly enhanced by the diet. The patient is on the road to remission.

With a positive attitude in operation, the chemical changes in the composition of the body have a greater effect. During periods of dietary modification and corporal purification, the internal milieu is altered. Fat is depleted from the organs, tissues, and blood; the pH of the body fluids is shifted to a more acid condition; various beneficial enzymes and substances are released into the bloodstream. These changes alone might be enough to create an inhospitable environment for the malignancy. Combined with a positive mental attitude and the chemicals of faith and hope, they can actually lead to remissions.

Since a proper macrobiotic diet is tailored to the individual and his or her specific form of cancer, it is impossible to present one unified program here. For a program that is right for you and your problem, contact a chapter of the East West Foundation or any other qualified counseling agency. In addition to the diet, they will provide tremendous personal support and advice and also an introduction to the philosophy behind the diet. This philosophy is an important part of the therapy, since it provides for the change in attitude that enhances the effects of the diet and brings you one step closer to remission.

If you can't get to a macrobiotic teacher right away but think you would benefit from this type of program, here are a few things you can do in the meantime to get yourself going in the right direction. First, read a recognized book on the subject. If this is difficult for you because of age, debility, or reading deficiency, get some help from a friend or family member who could explain some of the finer points. During this learning period, you can implement a change in your present diet by using the following recommendations as a simple introduction to macrobiotics:

- Eliminate all red meat from your diet. This includes not only steak and hamburger, but also breakfast and luncheon meats like bacon, sausage, and cold cuts.

- Significantly cut down on chicken and fish. (The more rigid macrobiotic diets require complete elimination of these foods, but as a transition to a meatless diet, they are acceptable in small quantities.)

- Eliminate all animal by-products, including lard, butter, cheese, and eggs.

- Replace animal proteins with the vegetables and vegetable juices of your choice. You can eat these in any quantity—the more the better—but you should prepare them without oil or butter. Mild seasonings are acceptable.

- Avoid sweet foods and sugar.

- Replace sweets with natural grains and cereals, occasionally fruits.

- Replace white flour with whole-grain products.

- Mix beans and vegetables for adequate protein intake.

- Use fresh foods in preference to canned or processed foods.

- Increase your consumption of pure water. In fact, replace other beverages with water or tea.

- For vitamin and mineral requirements, take a potent multivitamin and multimineral supplement each day.

These are just a few recommendations to help you make a smooth transition from your present diet to a macrobiotic diet, which must be structured around your individual illness and needs. You will need dedication and perseverance, but that is a small price to pay for your life.

A macrobiotic program can be your way of running the last lap against cancer and winning the race. It can be the powerful, life-saving factor you add to your standard medical or surgical treatment. Remember, too, a macrobiotic diet can be used effectively in conjunction with other self-directed therapies, particularly the nutritional supplementation program discussed in the following chapter.

Recommended Reading

Brown, V. *Macrobiotic Miracle*. New York: Japan Publications, 1984.

Heidenry, C. *An Introduction to Macrobiotics*. Brookline, MA: Aladdin Press, 1984.

Katzsch, R. *Macrobiotics Yesterday and Today*. New York: Japan Publications, 1985.

Kushi, M. *Cancer Prevention Diet*. New York: St. Martin's Press, 1983.

Kushi, M. and A. Kushi. *The Book of Macrobiotics*. Tokyo, Japan: Japan Publications, 1977.

Kushi, M. and R. Mendelsohn. *Cancer and Heart Disease*. New York: Japan Publications, 1982.

Nussbaum, E. *Recovery*. New York: Japan Publications, 1986.

Satillaro, A. *Recalled by Life*. Boston, MA: Houghton Mifflin, 1982.

MACROBIOTIC GUIDELINES

	PRIMARY FACTORS	CONTRIBUTING FACTORS	PROTECTIVE FACTORS
Bladder	Dairy products, eggs, fat, poultry, oil, red meat, white sugar	Air pollution, artificial sweeteners, chlorinated water, fruit, soft drinks, white flour	Beans, green and yellow vegetables, sea vegetables, spring water
Bone	Eggs, fat, meat, salt	Dairy products, radiation, stimulants, white sugar	Beans, shiitake mushrooms, sea salt, sea vegetables, whole grains
Brain (inner region)	Dairy products, eggs, oily fish, red meat	Drugs, fruit, juice, medications, oil, pesticides, stimulants, white sugar	Beans, sea vegetables, vegetables, whole grains
Brain (outer region)	Dairy products, drugs, chemicals, fats and oil, medication, soft drinks, spices, white sugar	Meat, synthetic clothing, vinyl chloride, other plastics	Beans, sea vegetables, vegetables, whole grains

MACROBIOTIC GUIDELINES

	PRIMARY FACTORS	CONTRIBUTING FACTORS	PROTECTIVE FACTORS
Breast	Dairy products, fats and oil, white flour and sugar	Drugs, eggs, meat and poultry, medication, soft drinks, spices	Beans, leafy green and white vegetables, soyfoods, whole grains
Endometrium	Dairy products, fats and oil, red meat, white flour and sugar	Birth-control pills, chemicals, estrogens, fruit	Beans, sea vegetables, vegetables, whole grains
Esophagus	Chemicals, dairy products, fats, oil, soft drinks, white sugar	Alcohol, meat—particularly cured (e.g., bacon, ham), radiation, tobacco	Beans, green and yellow vegetables, lentils, sea vegetables, whole grains
Kidney	Dairy products, fats, oil, red meat	Chemicals, drugs, fruit, juice, medication, soft drinks, stimulants, white sugar	Beans, sea vegetables, vegetables, whole grains
Large intestine (colon and rectum)	Eggs, fats, poultry, red meat	Beer, chemicals, dairy products, drugs, medication, oil, soft drinks, spices, white sugar	Beans and lentils, fiber, leafy green vegetables, sea vegetables, whole grains—and thorough chewing

MACROBIOTIC GUIDELINES

	PRIMARY FACTORS	CONTRIBUTING FACTORS	PROTECTIVE FACTORS
Leukemia	Chemicals, fats, oil, soft drinks, stimulants, white sugar	Animal food,* fruit, industrial pollutants, pesticides, radiation, spices, x-rays	Beans, miso, sea salt, sea vegetables, vegetables, whole grains
Liver	Animal food,* eggs, fats, oil, meat, white flour	Alcohol, birth-control pills, dairy products, drugs, medication, spices, white sugar	Beans, sea vegetables, shiitake mushrooms, vegetables, whole grains
Lung	Dairy products, eggs, oil, poultry and meat, white flour and sugar	Air pollution, asbestos, drugs, fruit, spices, stimulants, tobacco	Beans, leafy green and yellow vegetables, sea vegetables, whole grains, fresh air
Lymphoma and Hodgkin's disease	Chemicals, dairy, fats, oil, soft drinks, white sugar	Animal food,* benzene, pesticides, radiation, spices, tonsillectomies, x-rays	Beans, nuts, pulses, sea vegetables, seeds, vegetables, whole grains
Melanoma	Dairy products, eggs, oil, poultry and meat, white flour and sugar	Chemicals, fruit, medication, PCBs, soft drinks, spices, stimulants	Beans, sea vegetables, vegetables, whole grains

MACROBIOTIC GUIDELINES

	PRIMARY FACTORS	CONTRIBUTING FACTORS	PROTECTIVE FACTORS
Ovary	Animal food,* dairy products, eggs, fats, oil, meat	Birth-control pills, chemicals, fruit, juices, stimulants, white flour and sugar	Beans, sea vegetables, shiitake mushrooms, vegetables, whole grains
Pancreas	Cheese, eggs, fats, oil, poultry and meat, white sugar	Coffee, dairy products, radiation, spices, tobacco, white flour	Beans, sea vegetables, shiitake mushrooms, vegetables, whole grains
Prostate and testicles	Cheese, eggs, fats, meat	Chemicals, coffee, dairy products, drugs, fruit, medication, oil, white flour and sugar	Beans, sea vegetables, shiitake mushrooms, vegetables, whole grains
Skin	Chemicals, dairy products, fats and oil, fruit, juice, soft drinks, spices, white flour and sugar	Animal food*, industrial pollutants, sunlight	Beans, sea vegetables, soyfoods, sunlight plus low-fat diet, vegetables, whole grains
Stomach	Alcohol, oil, vinegar, white flour and rice	Animal food,* dairy products, industrial pollutants	Beans, leafy green and white vegetables, miso, sea vegetables, soyfoods, whole grains

*Animal food refers to any product that comes from animals: dairy products, meats and poultry, animal fats, blood, etc.

Adapted from *The Cancer Prevention Diet* by Michio Kushi. Copyright 1983 by Michio Kushi and Alex Jack. Used with permission from the publication, St. Martin's Press Inc, New York.

MACROBIOTIC CENTERS

Academy of the Healing
Arts
P.O. Box 31211
San Francisco, CA 94131

Center for Holistic Health
141 Fifth Avenue
New York, NY 10010

Community Health
Foundation
188 Old Street
London, EC1 England

East West Center
2525 West Gunnison Street
Chicago, IL 60625

East West Center
347 Ludlow Avenue
Cincinnati, OH 45220

East West Center
1013 Venus Road
Colorado Springs, CO
80906

East West Center
P.O. Box 1620
Fernie, B.C. Canada V0B
1M0

East West Center
P.O. Box 37
Forestville, CA 95436

East West Center
7511 Franklin Street
Hollywood, CA 90046

East West Center
2900 Torquay Road
Muncie, IN 47304

East West Center
142 West 44th Street
New York, NY 10023

East West Center
993 Portland Avenue
St. Paul, MN 55104

East West Center
2731 Fleetwood Drive
San Bruno, CA 94006

East West Center
264—A East Newton
Seattle, WA 98102

East West Center
10 Brook Avenue
Toronto, ON, Canada M5M
2J6

East West Center
696 West 20 Avenue
Vancouver, B.C. Canada
V5Z 1Y1

East West Center
32 Burncoat Street
Worcester, MA 01695

East West Foundation
6 Radcliff Road
Bala Cynwyd, PA 19004

East West Foundation
6209 Park Heights Avenue
Baltimore, MD 21215

East West Foundation
359 Boylston Street
Boston, MA 02116

East West Foundation
17 Station Street
Brookline, MA 02146

East West Foundation
3921 SW 60th Court
Miami, FL 33155

East West Foundation
P.O. Box 40012
Washington, DC 20016

Macrobiotic Guide to
  Natural Living
506A York Road
Towson, MD 21204

Macrobiotic Health Center
  of New Jersey
300 Washington Avenue
Belleville, NJ 07109

Vega Institute
P.O. Box 426
Oroville, CA 95965

8
Nutritional Supplementation and the Remission of Cancer

Unfortunately, the nutritional status of as many as half of all Americans is below acceptable standards. According to the U.S. Department of Agriculture, half of the population is daily deficient in some nutritional element, and our diets are getting worse every day. As a society on the go, we tend to eat on the run, stopping in fast-food restaurants more and more frequently. Consequently, the tendency is increasingly to eat fatty foods or foods that are deep-fried and dripping with oil. Worse yet, many people consume huge quantities of empty calories, foods that really have no nutritional value whatsoever, like candy, soda, white bread, and black coffee with sugar. All high in sugar or bleached white flour, these items deliver a punch that has no nutritional power.

Even when a diet appears acceptable, it may create hidden problems. For example, most farm crops are greatly depleted of nutritional value. The practice of growing single crops has caused farm soil to become minerally deficient, requiring heavy fertilization to sustain yields. The manufactured fertilizers used in the process are inorganic and incomplete; they deliver enough alimentation for growth but not for the nutritional value of the food. Furthermore, emphasizing speed of growth and size of crop has produced large, durable, and aesthetically appealing food, but these products are greatly devitalized and nutritionally inferior to previous harvests. Consumption of these foods is certainly better than eating junk food, but it still presents a problem for the person in need of an improved diet.

Even the concept of a minimum daily requirement is faulty. As children, we consumed more food per body weight than we do as adults, perhaps three to four times more. As our metabolism slows down with adulthood, it becomes more and more difficult to consume the necessary calories to deliver full nutritional requirements. To get all the vitamins and minerals needed for good health, we would have to eat so much food that obesity would eventually result. Indeed, this doom has befallen many individuals, with a disastrous impact on their health. Clearly, the sword has a double edge. To avoid the negative effects of too much food or too few vitamins, supplementation is the answer. To assist cancer patients who are in great need of supernutrition, supplementation is a must.

Nutritional supplementation is related to both metabolic and macrobiotic therapies. It encompasses the consumption of vitamins, minerals, and other nutrients with demonstrated value in strengthening the body, bolstering the immune system, and generally improving health. While the list of nutritional supplements is enormous, a few elements have particular benefit for the cancer patient. These include vitamins A, B_6 and C; folic and pantothenic acids; and enzymes and glandular extracts.

VITAMIN C

Perhaps the most beneficial, certainly the most acclaimed, nutritional supplement is vitamin C. Take a look at just a couple examples of its effectiveness.

In 1976 two well-known experts in the field of nutritional health conducted a vast study of the effects of vitamin C on patients with terminal cancer. Those men, Ewan Cameron from the Vale of Lebanon Hospital in Scotland and Linus Pauling of the Institute of Health and Science, closely followed 1,100 terminal cancer patients, 100 of whom were placed on high doses of vitamin C and 1,000 of whom were not. Otherwise, all conditions were similar, all treatments were alike, and all cases were classified as hopeless.

The results of their investigations were astounding. On the average, the patients who received the vitamin C lived four times longer than the larger control group. Sixteen of the 100 who received the vitamin C lived for over one year, while only three of the 1,000 survived for that period of time. (That's 16 percent of the vitamin C patients compared to less than 0.5 percent of the nonvitamin C group.) In addition, 12 of the patients who took the vitamin C completely recovered. All of the patients who did not receive the vitamin supplementation expired. It may seem incredible, but a substance as common as vitamin C had an overwhelmingly positive effect on the course and recovery of patients with terminal cancer.

Other benefits resulted as well. The vitamin C patients demonstrated a much better attitude than their control counterparts. They experienced better appetites and less pain. Some were even able to tolerate their discomfort without any pain medication at all, a feat that was impossible before the vitamin C supplementation. In retrospect, Dr. Pauling stated that the results could have been more impressive if he had administered higher doses of the vitamin. He believed that the cancer death rate could have been diminished by as much as 75 percent.

Just one year later, in 1977, scientific studies conducted on animal and human subjects found that antibodies circulating in the blood, tiny little protein structures that combine with and then destroy cancer cells, are more abundant in people with higher levels of vitamin C. Concurrent with the investigations that uncovered this important news, researchers also discovered that vitamin C was a necessary component in the process that produces an enzyme, C1 esterase, needed by the immune system to recognize foreign invaders in the body. Without this enzyme, cancer cells would go undetected, and their destruction would be much more difficult.

Vitamin C has been shown to have a tremendous effect on the immune system, particularly on white blood cells. Studies from the National Cancer Institute have demonstrated that the number of lymphocytes in the blood increases with increased intake of vitamin C. In fact, there is a direct association: the more vitamin C, the more lymphocytes. Apparently, the vitamin stimulates the actual production of these white blood cells, through the genesis of lymphoblasts—the immature bone marrow and lymph gland cells that give rise to lymphocytes. Additionally, vitamin C, along with zinc, linoleic acid, and pyridoxine, is required for the production of T lymphocytes, the cells that play such an important role in the identification of malignancies.

The activity of interferon, the antiviral, anticancer agent, is also enhanced by vitamin C. Scientists are not yet sure whether this action is caused by an increase in the number of interferon-producing cells or by a direct effect on the anticancer substance itself. Regardless, the enhancement was demonstrated in 1974 and 1975 by two prominent researchers, Drs. Schwerdt and Siegel, and reported in "Cancer and Vitamin C," a publication of the Institute of Health and Science in Menlo Park, California.

These are just two of many studies that have shown an astonishing correlation between nutritional supplementation and recovery from cancer. From investigations conducted in the United States to research projects undertaken in other parts of world, data have confirmed, time and time again, that nutritional augmentation is an important component of cancer therapy. Any health care professionals who think otherwise or advise their patients against daily supplementation are severely limited in their thinking and their knowledge. Not only do vitamins, minerals, and enzymes help to prevent cancers from developing, they also assist the body in the destruction and elimination of malignant disease once it has occurred.

VITAMIN B₆, PANTOTHENIC ACID, FOLIC ACID, AND VITAMIN A

Several other food supplements enhance the power of the immune system against cancer. Among them are vitamin B_6 and pantothenic and folic acids. According to studies from the University of Pittsburgh's school of medicine, and cited in Lynn Dallin's *Cancer Causes and Natural Controls*, absence of these individual nutritional elements would greatly compromise the effectiveness of the immune system because there would be no circulating antibodies. Expressed in another way, vitamin B_6, pantothenic acid, and folic acid are absolutely necessary for production of the antibodies that eliminate cancer.

In addition to their ability to stimulate the immune system and participate in certain biological reactions that produce immune cells and the products of those cells, nutritional supplements appear to have a direct deleterious effect on tumor cells. According to research by Michael Sporn at the National Cancer Institute, substances similar to vitamin A help to maintain cell maturity, thus preventing cells from reverting back to immature forms that are characteristic of cancer. Vitamin A itself, along with selenium and vitamin E—all classified as antioxidants—have a possible role in the disruption of the respiratory process of malignant cells. Dr. Sporn hypothesizes that these three nutritional components act in a way that makes cancer cells unable to "breathe" in a manner that allows them to produce the energy they need to grow and divide. Without this capability, they cannot survive.

This theory is partially supported by research from the Cleveland Clinic. Following the completion of several investigations, researchers concluded that vitamin A not only hinders the formation of cancer cells, but that it impedes their growth. Exactly how this inhibition occurs is the continuing topic of numerous ongoing projects. The limitation of malignant cell respiration is a definite possibility, considering the known characteristics of the antioxidants.

ENZYMES

Another group of supplements that receives high acclaim and enthusiastic recommendation from holistic physicians is the collection of enzymes produced by the pancreas. According to metabolic doctors, cancer patients lack these enzymes for two reasons. Either the pancreas itself is an inadequate producer, or the enzymes are completely used up in the digestion of protein from an overly protein-rich diet. In each case, supply is inadequate for anticancer activities.

Even when the quantity of pancreatic enzymes is normal, extenuating circumstances may prevent proper use. For instance, when vitamin deficiencies exist, enzymes cannot function properly. They all require a full complement of vitamins, which act as chemical catalysts—substances that speed up enzymatic reactions and allow them to go to chemical completion. Without vitamins to act as chemical assistants, enzymes fail to perform their functions properly. Like bombs without fuses, their potential cannot be realized, and their anti-cancer qualities are lost.

The importance of enzymatic action against cancer has been observed since the turn of the century. In the late 1800s, enzymes were applied to ulcerated cancer wounds with positive results. Later, European doctors experimented with enzyme therapies and found them to be of great value in the general treatment of cancer. Apparently, the pancreatic enzymes weaken malignant cell walls and enhance the action of natural defense cells and their antibodies. With a decrease in the integrity of the cell wall, the entire cancer cell becomes more vulnerable to the action of specific therapeutic and natural forces.

At the Wolf Zimmer Clinic in Germany, a comprehensive study was undertaken to determine the combined effect of radiation therapy used in conjunction with enzyme treatments. Conducted in the early 1960s, this study showed that a high proportion, two out of every three patients, responded positively. This response rate was significantly higher than that achieved with radiation alone. Similar results have been drawn from a host of international research projects over the past 25 years.

Today, holistic doctors regularly treat their cancer patients with various pancreatic enzymes and, according to their reports, firmly believe that enzymes are the most important form of supplementation a patient can receive. They are convinced that enzymes have a more noticeable effect on malignancies than any other form of supplementation but also maintain that all enzymes must be used with copious amounts of other nutrients, specifically, vitamins and minerals. In addition, they advise patients to constantly cleanse the body of the toxins that result from dead and dying tumor cells, the result of enzyme action. This cleansing is accomplished through various techniques described in the chapter on metabolic therapies—treatments like liver and gall-bladder purges, kidney flushes, and coffee enemas. These measures not only help to ensure total health, they also increase the effectiveness of the treatments.

GLANDULAR EXTRACTS

An additional and final component of a total nutritional supplementation program is consumption of glandular extracts. These extracts are ground-up whole organ concentrates that are compressed into pill or capsule form. Once ingested and absorbed, they are directly incorporated into the corresponding bodily organ (the liver or adrenals, for example), where they help to support the functions of each particular organ. For example, liver extract is absorbed by the intestines and is assimilated into the living tissue of the liver. Since this incorporation is a gradual process, the ingestion of liver extract, like all other supplements, must be ongoing. Over time, the liver will function more effectively because it will have all the necessary ingredients to do so. The same is true of the adrenals, the pancreas, the thyroid, and the thymus gland—perhaps the most important gland in the treatment of cancer.

Present thinking suggests that the most important glandular extract is that from the thymus—the lymph gland that makes such an important contribution to the formation of the immune system. During infancy and childhood, the thymus produces an abundant supply of T lymphocytes that migrate to the other lymph glands of the body and set up colonies of similar cells. As the thymus recedes with age, the cells that it produced and left behind continue to protect the body from enemy invaders, like cancer. They also continue to respond to stimulation from a variety of sources, including glandular extracts from ground thymus tissue. This outside stimulation increases the number of T cells, and each cell is brought to a higher degree of readiness and potency. Stronger in number and power, they can more adequately defend the body from deleterious forces and can improve the chances of surviving a dreaded illness like cancer.

The vitamins, minerals, enzymes, and glandular extracts just discussed form the basis for a supplementation program that has a twofold purpose: (1) to strengthen the immune system by increasing the number and effectiveness of immune cells and their anticancer by-products; and (2) to directly inhibit cancer cells themselves. By implementing such a program, the cancer patient assists the body in its attempt to retard and reverse the cancerous process. At the same time, the patient will realize improved overall health by supplying the essential ingredients for normal bodily functions.

It is also important to note that general good health, facilitated by a blend of *all* necessary nutrients, can aid in the dissipation of cancer.

COMMON FOODS WITH ANTICANCER QUALITIES

Just as certain foods have been shown to increase the chances of developing cancer, others have demonstrated anticancer qualities. As a specific example, *Health* magazine reported that the researcher, Dr. Tariq Abdullah of the Akbar Clinic and Research Center, has shown that common garlic offers significant benefit to cancer patients, adding substance to the old wives' tale that the small but mighty bulbs can, indeed, fight malignancies. According to reports from the Panama City, Florida Clinic, garlic more than doubles the potency of natural killer cells, those powerful lymphocytes that destroy cancer cells but leave normal cells unharmed. Dr. Abdullah comments that the cause of the lymphocyte enhancement is unknown but the benefit is nonetheless real and documented. He further remarks that the power is in fresh, not cooked, garlic.

As reported in Dallin's book, *Cancer Causes and Natural Controls*, other foods found to be beneficial are those high in vitamin and mineral content—fresh green vegetables in general and those rich in chlorophyll in particular. Asparagus, for example, receives high acclaim by cancer-conscious groups. The interest in this vegetable began when a Pittsburgh dentist claimed to have cured his lymph and eye cancers with its use. Later, Karl B. Lutz, a retired chemist, collected fifty cases of asparagus cures attributed to the high folic acid, nucleic acid, and histone levels in the vegetable. Additionally, Emanuel Rivici, director of the Institute of Applied Biology in New York, points out that methyl mercaptan, a substance secreted into the urine following the ingestion of asparagus, has distinct anticancer qualities.

As an example of a food high in enzymes, papaya is known to contain numerous substances that break down scar tissue and tumorous growths. Its enzymes have been shown to work well in acid, alkaline, and neutral environments, and Eastern nutritionists have rated it the best of all foods. For more specific information about individual foods and their anticancer potentials, you might want to read *Cancer Causes and Natural Controls* by Lynn Dallin.

SUPPLEMENTATION SCHEDULE

On a serious supplementation program, items are taken literally around the clock. The first consumption occurs early in the morning, when the body is most alkaline and the cells are most susceptible. Usually at this time, a host of pancreatic enzymes are consumed. These include two powerful digestive supplements known as trypsin and chymotrypsin, each of which may have a role in weakening the external walls of cancer cells.

Just before breakfast, the second group of supplements is taken. This group includes a variety of minerals, especially those most crucially needed by the individual patient. Their consumption is critical to the proper completion of the biochemical reactions that drive the body, reactions required for enzymes to function correctly and for the normal processes of the body to take place. Also at this time, the glandular extracts are consumed. As you have seen, these supplements are used to stimulate their corresponding organs to perform as effectively as possible.

Additional supplementation occurs during meals, with the ingestion of more vitamins, minerals, and enzymes. This is necessary because the absorption of vitamins and minerals usually requires the assistance of various components in whole food. For example, some form of fat must be present in the intestines for the complete absorption of the fat-soluble vitamins. Likewise, vitamin D and calcium absorption are linked.

The enzymes taken with meals help to digest the food, thereby diminishing the dependency on internal enzymes and reserving them for direct anticancer activities. Enzymes are again taken in midafternoon, when the metabolism of the body nears its daily peak and the body fluids again become comparatively alkaline.

Finally, the last round of supplements for the day occurs shortly before bedtime. This consumption consists of calcium, magnesium, and tryptophan—substances that calm the body and lead to a relaxed state conducive to sleep. The importance of this supplementation is not its potential effect on the cancer, but rather its effect on the patient's relaxation. Sleep is extremely beneficial in the recovery from all illnesses and should not be overlooked in the treatment of cancer.

Considerations in Planning a Supplementation Program

While the ingestion of adequate amounts of vitamins, minerals, enzymes, and extracts is important in the maintenance of good health and the recovery from illness, an anticancer diet can be of great benefit, too. Try to combine both forms of treatment into one overall program that includes the proper use of nutritional supplements as well as a strong macrobiotic diet. Critics have pointed out that while the macrobiotic diet is powerfully therapeutic, it unfortunately lacks many of the vitamins and minerals essential for the proper functioning of the body. To gain the benefits of such a diet and still maintain adequate nutrition, take supplements. In doing so, the prudent approach is to seek professional guidance to design an appropriate program combining these two therapies.

If you decide to participate in a real supplementation program, seek out professional guidance before initiating any homemade plan of supernutrition. Too often, a well-meaning patient will begin a program unaided, without the proper knowledge to augment it well. Incorrect amounts and unsuitable combinations of vitamins, minerals, and enzymes are the unfortunate result, leading to an inadequate and unacceptable outcome. At times the results can be downright disastrous, actually jeopardizing rather than benefiting the patient's health. The wise approach to this and any other form of self-administered therapy is to obtain the advice of professionals who work with the subject every day. This approach generates the best program and the best results.

With the decision to begin a program of supplementation comes the responsibility to maintain that program with dedication and persistence. Like all of the other forms of adjunct, self-directed treatments, supplementation must become a normal part of your day. It must become habit. You must view it as a part of your treatment that is essential to your recovery. As such, you must continue it uninterruptedly and indefinitely.

Recommended Reading

Adams, R. and F. Murray. *Improving Your Health with Vitamin C*. New York: Larchmont Books, 1978.

Cameron, E., and L. Pauling. *Cancer and Vitamin C.* Menlo Park, CA: Linus Pauling Institute of Science and Medicine, 1979.

Cheraskin, E. and W.M. Ringsdorf. *New Hope for Incurable Disease.* New York: Arco, 1971.

Dallin, L. *Cancer Causes and Natural Controls.* Port Washington, NY: Ashley Books Inc., 1983.

Mayer, J. *A Diet for Living,* New York: Pocket Books, 1977.

Mindell, E. *Vitamin Bible,* New York: Rawson-Wade, 1979.

Newbold, H. L. *Vitamin C Against Cancer.* New York: Stein & Day, 1981.

Passwater, R. A. *Cancer and Its Nutritional Therapies.* New Canaan, CT: Pivot Original Health Books, 1978.

———. *Supernutrition: Megavitamin Revolution.* New York: Pocket Books, 1976.

———. *Supernutrition.* New York: Dial Press, 1975.

Pfeiffer, C. C. *Zinc and Other Micro-Nutrients.* New Canaan, CT: Keats Publishing, 1978.

Pritikin, N. *The Pritikin Promise: 28 Days to a Longer, Healthier Life.* New York: Simon and Schuster, 1983.

Shute, W. E. *The Complete Updated Vitamin E Book.* New Canaan, CT: Keats Publishing, 1975.

Stone, I. *The Healing Factor: Vitamin C Against Disease.* New York: Grosset & Dunlap, 1972.

Williams, R. J. *Nutrition Against Disease.* New York: Pitman, 1971.

NUTRITION FOUNDATIONS, CENTERS, AND INSTITUTES

American Nutritional
  Medical Association
1326 Dearborn Street
Gary, IN 46403

Atlantic Nutritional
  Association
1301 Massachusetts
  Avenue, NW
Suite 703
Washington, DC 20005

Coalition for Alternatives
in Nutrition and Health
Care
P.O. Box B-12
Richlandtown, PA 18955

International College of
Applied Nutrition
Referral Service
312 East Las Tunas Drive
San Gabriel, CA 91776

National Herbalist
Foundation
271 Fifth Avenue
New York, NY 10016

Natural Food Associates
P.O. Box 210
Atlanta, TX 75551

Network for Better
Nutrition
2910 Brandy Wine Street,
NW
Washington, DC 20008

North American Nutrition
and Preventive Medicine
Association
P.O. Box 592
Colony Square Station
Atlanta, GA 30361

Nutrition Education
Association
3647 Glen Haven
Houston, TX 77025

Nutrition for Optimal
Health Association
P.O. Box 380
Winnetka, IL 60093

Nutrition Today Society
703 Giddings Avenue
Annapolis, MD 21404

Price Pottenger Nutrition
Foundation
P.O. Box 2614
La Mesa, CA 92041

NUTRITION AND SUPPLEMENTATION PHYSICIANS AND CLINICS

Ray Beach, D.C.
300 West 23rd St.
Freemont, NE 68025
402-721-1190

Lauri Campbell, N.D.
12027 Arbour St.
Windsor, ON N8N 1N7
Canada
519-735-1384

Michael Cessna, D.C.
504 North 13th Street
Rogers, AR 72756
501-636-1178

Ruth Cilento, M.D.
1 Trackson Street
Alderley, Brisbane, 4051
Australia 07-352-6634

John Cosh, M.D.
Cancer Help Centre
Grove House, Cornwallis
Grove
Clifton, Bristol BS8 4PG
England
0272 743216

Linus Pauling Institute
440 Page Mill Road
Palo Alto, CA 94306
415-327-4064

Ruth Yale Long, Ph.D.
3647 Glen Haven
Houston, TX 77025
713-665-2946

James Privitera, M.D.
105 North Grandview
Covina, CA 91723
818-966-1618

Dorothea Snook, N.D.
Radiant Health Centre
Private Hospital
Doctor's Hill
Northam, West Australia

9
Exercise and the Remission of Cancer

He's one of the longest-living survivors of what is perhaps the worst of all illnesses: AIDS. He has carried the diagnosis for over six years and is still doing well. Averting all of AIDS's symptoms and avoiding the progression to Kaposi's sarcoma, a devastating form of cancer, he has kept himself together with the physical exertion of a rigid and vigorous daily exercise program. He's young, energetic, and determined. His life's goal is to keep on living.

Although he will remain anonymous in this discussion, this patient is well known among AIDS researchers, causing current reports on AIDS to be rewritten, providing undeniable proof that the disease is not always rapidly fatal and that there is, indeed, hope for all AIDS sufferers. This hope comes in many forms, one of which is exercise.

The course of cancer, like that of AIDS and many other illnesses, is affected by a number of factors, primary of which is the physical condition of the patient.

As a degenerative and progressive disease, cancer worsens or improves depending on the weakness or strength of the mind and body. Its progress almost exactly parallels the status of the immune system and the competence of the cells and chemicals that compose that system. Therefore, for the individual who carries the diagnosis of cancer, AIDS, or any other serious medical malady, it is imperative to remain as healthy as possible and to do everything possible to bolster the immune response to illness.

That's the purpose of a complete, well-rounded, and scientific exercise program. It not only strengthens the bones and muscles, the heart and lungs, it also increases the potency of the immune system and literally makes every cell in the body function better. That includes the white blood cells, which are essential in the fight against cancer.

RESEARCH INTO THE BENEFITS OF EXERCISE

According to James Ewing, who researched and reported on cancer nearly seventy-five years ago, the highest occurrence of malignancy at the time his report was concluded was among the physically inactive—people who were either unable or unwilling to physically exert themselves. A few years later, in 1921, a comprehensive study of approximately 86,000 cancer patients revealed that the highest death rates in the group were among patients who were the least physically active. The same observations are seen in many other similar studies and confirm the benefit of maintaining the highest possible level of fitness in order to better fight disease.

Animal experiments reveal the same sort of results. Perhaps the most intriguing study of all, conducted by Drs. Paschkis and Hoffman, followed the progress of tumor growth in laboratory mice. The two scientists discovered that reduced tumor growth and even the complete reversal of malignancy occurred when diseased mice were injected with an extract taken from healthy mice that had just been exercised to the point of exhaustion. This particular study is of great interest because it proved several important points. Most significantly, it showed that cancer can be reversed. Next, it proved that special chemicals are released by the body during periods of vigorous exercise. And finally, it demonstrates that these chemicals, whatever they may be, are responsible for the reversal of cancerous tumor growth.

Although the results of animal research studies only hint at possible correlations in humans, we know from research into human physiology that similar conditions exist in our own bodies. Take for instance the release of endorphins, those magical chemicals emitted from the brain. The release begins during periods of physical activity. From the brain, endorphins continue to circulate throughout the body for hours, performing their miracles wherever they are needed.

Of course, many other beneficial changes occur within the body during periods of vigorous exercise. From the studies of Kenneth Cooper in the early 1960s, we have learned that good exercises, those that expand the cardiovascular capacity, not only benefit the heart and lungs, but bring the rest of the body to a much better state of overall health. Higher demand for oxygen during physical activity causes blood vessels to expand throughout the body in order to deliver more oxygenated blood. The resultant increase in blood flow greatly benefits the cancer patient because the cells and chemicals of the immune system must also travel in the bloodstream. As the delivery of these anticancer agents improves, so does the effect they have on the tumor.

Effective exercise speeds up the metabolic processes, including digestion, absorption, and elimination. Consequently, the incorporation of beneficial nutrients into body tissues is greatly enhanced, as is the elimination of toxins through the liver, skin, and kidneys. In addition, the benefits of all the metabolic therapies soon to be discussed are substantially increased. Exercise lowers resting cardiac and respiratory rates, thereby conserving the energy needed by cancer patients to fight their illnesses. And exercise improves mental attitude, providing patients with tremendous psychological strength. All in all, it is one of the most positive and beneficial therapies that can be initiated in an adjunct program.

But is it OK for cancer patients to exert themselves vigorously in a daily exercise program? Or is it better for them to rest and try to slowly recover from their illness? Of course, rest is important for everyone, especially for someone who suffers from cancer. Extreme fatigue and total exhaustion should be avoided. But there are no reasons for cancer patients to avoid exercise and many reasons why they should participate. According to Carl Simonton, whose work with visualization and cancer is discussed later in this book, cancer patients can perform almost any kind of exercise and can function at almost the same level as they did before their illness was diagnosed. Many patients, in fact, actually function at higher levels of physical exertion after participating in an exercise routine that builds strength and endurance. Some patients have even entered marathon races and competitive sports with positive results and no ill effects. Simonton also points out that patients who do implement a daily exercise program become healthier, more self-sufficient and confident, exhibiting less vulnerability and depression. They develop a mental attitude that carries with it a better prognosis for their illness.

Of all the exercises that can be performed by cancer patients, or by anyone for that matter, aerobic exercises are the best. Those who are unfamiliar with the term *aerobic* should pick up a copy of Kenneth Cooper's fabulous book *Aerobics* and use it as a reference and guide. It contains not only an explanation of the concept of aerobic exercise, but also an entire program around which you can tailor your own daily routine.

Generally, aerobic exercises are those that increase the body's demand for oxygen. They include running and jogging, swimming, walking, cycling, and competitive sports like handball, racquetball, squash, and basketball that require a significant amount of nonstop activity and movement. As the exercise is performed, the body's energy requirements increase, and more oxygen is needed to fulfill those requirements. Consequently, the lungs work harder to breathe in more oxygen, and the heart beats faster to pump that oxygen throughout the body. The benefit of all this activity on overall health is impressive, including stronger heart and lungs; lower blood pressure; decreased levels of blood sugar, triglycerides, and cholesterol; better circulation; formation of new blood vessels; stronger metabolism; and a healthier immune system.

Dr. Cooper found the personal results of aerobic exercise on his patients to be simply remarkable. The obese lost weight. Smokers gave up cigarettes. The overly anxious calmed down. Recognizable introverts became more extroverted. Lung ailments disappeared. Ulcers healed. Diabetics reduced or completely eliminated their medication. While specific studies on exercise and cancer have never been properly undertaken, many research physicians including Cooper believe that increased physical activity, in the form of an aerobic exercise program, is invaluable. In fact, metabolic physicians and major health centers around the country, including Simonton's, Pritikin's, and Menninger's recommend exercise as part of their therapeutic regimen.

GUIDELINES FOR STARTING AN EXERCISE PROGRAM

The following guidelines for a general exercise program fit within the recommendations of Dr. Cooper and other experts in the field of exercise physiology. Use them as the basis for your own personal program by choosing sports and activities you particularly enjoy.

Choose an exercise that has good aerobic potential. Consider any from this group: running, jogging, walking, swimming, cycling, stationary jogging, stationary cycling, rowing, rope skipping, skiing, skating. Appropriate competitive sports include basketball, hockey, handball, racquetball, squash, and wrestling. Other common social games like golfing with a cart, tennis, and volleyball are certainly enjoyable but provide so little aerobic benefit that they are not included in the list.

Perform your exercise(s) at least every other day, but preferably every day. Cooper found that intermittent exercise did not increase endurance or fitness to any great extent. He also showed that any gains achieved with a specific routine were quickly lost if the patient abandoned the routine or followed it only partially. To be beneficial, exercise must be performed regularly.

During the activity, you must increase your heart rate to 75 percent of the maximum for your age. This is considered your aerobic target zone. Each of us has a standard resting heart rate, which is usually around 80 beats per minute. We also have a maximum rate, which ranges from 150 to 200 beats per minute depending on our age. (The older you are, the lower your maximum rate.) During periods of physical exertion, the demand on the heart increases, and so does the heart rate. As you continue to exercise, pushing yourself further all the time, your heart will continue to beat faster until it reaches a maximum level. Exercising at the maximum rate is like driving your car at full speed. Sooner or later, something's got to give.

So exercise instructors have devised a set of guidelines for safe yet effective conditioning. These include the recommendation to exercise at only 75 percent of maximum capacity, thereby reducing the possibility of

erious injury. The following chart lists the correct aer-
bic target rates for different ages.

AGE	BEATS PER MINUTE
20	150
30	140
40	130
50	120
60	110
70	. 100

You determine your heart rate during your exercise
essions just as a doctor would in his office—by taking
our pulse. You simply cease your activity for a moment, take a six-second pulse (count the number of
beats in six seconds), then multiply by ten to get the
beats per minute. If you are below the proper target
zone, increase the intensity of your exercise. If you are
above your target zones, slow down. It's easy and scientific, and you will never overexert yourself with this
method.

According to Cooper's original work, during each session, you must maintain your target rate, nonstop, for
at least twelve consecutive minutes. In thousands of test
subjects, Cooper showed that only twelve consecutive
minutes at the proper aerobic target zone increased endurance and fitness. Less than twelve minutes was insufficient, and more than twelve minutes was unnecessary. But twelve minutes of proper aerobic activity at
least every other day brought on all the wonderful results available from an exercise program. (Recently
Cooper has upgraded these recommendations and suggests an average of fifteen to twenty minutes per session.)

Follow the established recommendations of all
graded exercise programs by beginning the activity
with a gradual warm-up and ending it with a slow cool-

down period. This is really quite easy. It simply means
that before jogging, let's say, walk for a few minutes, or
perform stretching exercises, to warm up and loosen up
a bit. Then, after jogging, walk a little more to allow
your heart rate to gradually return to its resting level.
The same principles apply to all forms of exercise and
ensure the safety of the workout.

These rules represent only the core of an aerobic exercise program and must be expanded with information from more complete sources. Once you have chosen
your adjunct therapies, it's up to you to learn as much as
possible about each of them, so that you can perform
them with the highest degree of skill. You can use the
knowledge to intensify your fight and better your
chances against your illness.

You should, of course, inform your personal physician
of your intentions. Before starting, obtain an exercise
prescription from your doctor or a physical therapist.
This just makes good sense. If you have already been
exercising, you probably won't need an exercise prescription, but you should at least apprise your doctor
that you want to increase your activity as part of a self-
directed adjunct to the traditional therapies you are
receiving.

Recommended Reading

Bachman, D. C., and M. Preston. *Dear Dr. Jock: The People's
Guide to Sports and Fitness.* New York: Dutton, 1980.

Cantu, R. C. *Towards Fitness: Guided Exercises for Those
with Health Problems.* New York: Human Sciences Press
1980.

Chapian, M. *Fun to Be Fit: Staying in Shape with a Life
Changing Exercise Plan.* Old Tappan, NJ: Revell, 1983.

Cooper, K. H. *Aerobics.* New York: Bantam, 1980.

———. *The Aerobics Way.* New York: Bantam, 1978.

———. *The Aerobics Program for Total Well-Being: Exercise
Diet, Emotional Balance.* New York: Evans, 1982.

Fixx, J. *The Complete Book of Running.* New York: Random House, 1977.

Gilmore, C. P. *Exercising for Fitness.* Alexandria, VA: Time-Life Books, 1981.

Kuntzleman, C. T. and the Editors of *Consumer Guide. Rating the Exercises.* New York: Penguin, 1980.

Marchetti, A. *Dr. Marchetti's Walking Program.* New York: Stein & Day, 1980.

Marshall, J. L. *The Sports Doctor's Fitness Book for Women.* New York: Delacorte, 1981.

Sheehan, G. A. *Dr. George Sheehan's Medical Advice to Runners.* Mountain View, CA: World Publications, 1978.

Solomon, N. and E. Harrison. *Doctor Solomon's Proven Master Plan for Total Body Fitness and Maintenance.* New York: Berkley, 1978.

Spino, D. *New Age Training for Fitness and Health.* New York: Grove, 1979.

HEALTH CLUBS AND SPAS

For a complete list of health clubs and spas across the United States and elsewhere, consult:

Babcock, J. and J. Kennedy. *The Spa Book: A Guided, Personal Tour of Health Resorts and Beauty Spas for Men and Women.* New York: Crown, 1983.

Deitrich, J. and S. Waggoner. *The Complete Health Club Handbook.* New York: Simon and Schuster, 1983.

Schnirring, M. *The Well-Being Guide to Health Spas in North America.* New York: Atheneum, 1982.

Wilkens, E. More Secrets from the Super Spas. *New York* (December 1983): 207.

III
YOUR MENTAL
HEALER

10
Meditation and the Remission of Cancer

The patient, a young Australian, first noted a small black mole on the skin of his thigh and sought out medical assistance when the lesion suddenly enlarged and started to ulcerate and bleed. Upon examining the young man, his physicians diagnosed the problem as malignant melanoma and immediately removed the cancer by surgically excising the tumor along with a wide margin of skin to ensure total elimination. The doctors thought they had "got it all," but within eighteen months, the patient returned to the hospital for treatment of swollen glands in his groin—glands that contained cancer.

At this time, additional surgery was performed. A large area of skin, muscle, and connective tissue was removed from the groin in a procedure known as a block dissection. The intent is to try to eradicate the cancer by cutting out all the lymph glands and surrounding soft tissue in the region of the metastasis. Since the cancer originally started on the thigh, the first area of spread would be the lymph nodes of the groin. These clearly were already involved and had to be totally removed if the young man was to survive. The surgery was successfully performed and the patient was put on immunotherapy with BCG—an immune-system stimulator—in the hope of eradicating any other possible areas of involvement.

Unfortunately, another area developed. With signs of lung involvement—cough and discomfort—the patient returned to the hospital for further evaluation. A chest film was ordered, and in his lungs for all to see was yet another metastatic lesion, this one about the size of an apricot pit.

Treatment of this tumor would be difficult. First of all, it was considered to be inoperable, so surgery was definitely out. The BCG had proved ineffective, so it was discontinued. Chemotherapy and radiation were thought to be of marginal value in this case, so these two modes of therapy were not employed. Really, there was nothing more that anyone could do.

Luckily, the patient didn't sit around waiting. Under the watchful eye of Dr. Ainslie Meares of Melbourne, Australia, he was instructed in a program of intense meditation. "He learned to meditate easily," reported Dr. Meares, "and although still in full-time employment, averaged around two and a half hours of meditation daily." Through constant attention and continued meditation, the patient began to improve.

Within two months after the patient had initiated meditation, the radiologist who had been following the case reported that the tumor had shrunk; it was now only one-sixteenth of its original size. Subsequent x-rays revealed that the tumor had completely disappeared. Without any additional treatments with drugs, radiation, or surgery, the young Australian had saved his own life through a dedicated daily program of intense meditation. No other explanation could account for the dramatic turn of events in this wonderful case. The meditation had saved his life.

In a similar case, a thirty-five-year-old woman had a melanoma excised from her calf and at the same time had a block dissection of the groin performed for obvious metastases. Although she tolerated both procedures well, within two months she returned to the hospital for a recurrence of the cancer in her groin. Now her condition was much more discomforting. With the recurrence of cancer comes a poorer prognosis. And since the malignancy recurred at a site of metastases already unsuccessfully treated, the course of the disease was considered much worse. The patient was understandably anxious.

While therapeutics were being considered, the woman was referred for meditation to alleviate her anxiety. She began a daily program and progressed well in reducing the stress and worry associated with her grave prognosis. Miraculously, she progressed in other areas as well.

Within just three weeks of the commencement of meditation, the metastatic tumor in her groin began to undergo unusual changes. Initially, the skin over the area of resection thickened and hardened. Her doctors thought this change might represent a rapid proliferation of the malignant cells, so they viewed it as yet another negative sign and advised BCG therapy. But the young woman refused, opting instead for the meditation as sole therapy.

With her continued effort to meditate daily came another unusual change in the appearance of the metastatic lesion. Two weeks after the thickening developed, it mysteriously and spontaneously disappeared. Surprised and excited by this outcome, the woman furthered her personal effort and, much to the astonishment of her original physicians and herself, went into complete and permanent remission shortly thereafter.

The cases just presented are only two from a file of many remissions associated with meditation. They amply show that the effects of meditation on illness can be profound and that patients can take matters into their own hands to favorably influence the course of a disease.

MEDITATION AND PHYSICAL CHANGES

Meditation is a means of directing the attention of the mind that produces simultaneous and dramatic physical changes in the body, changes that can alter the internal environment just enough to make it inhospitable to malignant growth.

The first serious studies of the field of meditation occurred in the mid 1930s, when the French cardiologist Thérèse Brosse went to India with the thought of recording the remarkable claims of yogi meditators who supposedly could exist for extended periods of time in airtight containers and even stop their hearts from beating. Armed with a portable electrocardiograph, she monitored the physical effects of meditation and proved that the feats previously mentioned did indeed occur. She actually found a subject who could stop and restart his heart at will with absolutely no adverse repercussions.

Further work was done by Drs. Wanger and Bagchi of the Universities of California and Michigan. They too proved that yogis could consciously reduce their heart and respiratory rates by meditating and concentrating on the desired results. In the 1950s and 1960s researchers demonstrated that Zen monks in Japan could not only alter individual organ function, but could also lower their entire metabolic rate, effectively reducing oxygen consumption and carbon dioxide elimination. These results were also confirmed by the staff at the All-India Institute of Medical Sciences in New Delhi.

From the reports collected at the time, it appeared that the process of meditation exerted its remarkable effects on the body through the involuntary pathways of the autonomic nervous system—the system that acts in the transmission of stress from the conscious and unconscious mind to the physical body. As we've seen, more recent evidence suggested that the reverse process could take place. The mind could positively affect the body in ways that might have therapeutic benefit.

Another physical change noted by the initial investigators was the increase in skin resistance to an electrical current. This particular alteration had previously been associated with the reduction of anxiety, while a decrease in skin resistance seemed to reflect an increase in physical tension. It therefore appeared that meditation produced a profound state of relaxation and a decrease in stress.

From the patterns that developed over the course of many years in experiments too numerous to mention here, it become apparent that meditation generates a reflex response that acts through the central nervous system. The entire response is similar to the fight-or-flight reaction first described by Walter B. Cannon, the Harvard physiologist, except that it represents the reverse of Dr. Cannon's observations. Instead of increasing the heart rate, blood pressure, blood flow, and oxygen consumption, it actually lowers them. In effect, the meditation response is the exact opposite of the fight-or-flight reaction. As a reversal of this process, its application in medicine became apparent.

The forms of meditation that are currently practiced in the Western world stem basically from Zen meditation, as described by Alan Watts, and from the Transcendental Meditation of Maharishi Mahesh Yogi. Both of these forms of meditation are appropriate for therapeutic considerations, since each can produce a deep state of mental and physical relaxation. They are both characterized by the familiar EEG patterns of alpha brain wave activity and appear to be equally potent in their ability to alter cardiac and pulmonary functions.

Meditation as it is discussed here is not to be confused with simple contemplation or the mere deliberation on a thought or idea. It is the actual direction of attention.

It is an exercise that requires both learning and practice to perfect.

Also avoid associating the process with any particular faith, belief system, or group. Although meditation was introduced relatively recently to the West and popularized during the 1960s, it is a legitimate activity that has been practiced for centuries in Eastern societies. It should not be blindly identified with any particular person or event that might create a predrawn negative opinion of the merit of the exercise. Meditation is simply a way of focusing the mind to function in a specific fashion, a way of removing the constant chatter of conscious thinking in order to provide an avenue for the perception of the true self. While this may sound foreign or exotic, it is by no means unnatural. Researchers and participants alike have shown that meditation is as natural as any other learned function, as normal as any other form of mental activity.

While the goal of meditation—mastery of the attention, awareness of all internal stimuli, and an unobstructed flow of pure consciousness—might seem simple enough, it is not so easily obtained. Your mind is willful, so your attempts to rule your thoughts and quiet your constant mental turnings will encounter strong resistance. Your mind will want to jump from one topic to another, from one thought to the next. Your job is to arrest this incessant and involuntary activity and take control. With practice and persistence, you will master your mind and increase your ability to control your attention.

From the onset, you will notice the beneficial results that come with the practice of meditation. Most obvious will be the reduction of tension and anxiety. According to meditators and numerous research studies, meditation is physiologically more refreshing than natural sleep. Although EEG readings indicate it is associated with a completely different state of mind than that of sleep, it is considered to be regenerative and rejuvenating. In fact, most meditators report that they actually require less sleep each night when they are actively meditating. This finding seems to be particularly common among new practitioners and suggests that immediate benefit is derived from the activity.

In short order, additional, more profound changes begin to take place. A decrease in heart and respiratory rates will occur more frequently and intensely. Blood pressure will decline to excellent levels, and the natural immunity will improve. All of these changes enhance physical well-being and improve general health. More importantly to reversing the process that generates and sustains cancer, the chemical composition of the body will actually change.

According to Dr. Meares, "It seems likely that a number of different psychophysiological responses are called into play by intense meditation. The general reduction in the habitual level of anxiety reduces cortisol with consequent freeing of the immune system to act more effectively against cancer." As discussed in previous chapters, the mind-body connection that turns life events into stressful physical conditions is in large part related to the activity of the pituitary gland and the release of cortisol from the adrenal glands. More than any other substance produced by the body, cortisol has the most negative effect on the immune system, effectively reducing white blood cells in the thymus and lymph glands, reducing T helper and associated cells, inhibiting natural killer cells, and even reducing the amount of available interferon. These are precisely the conditions that cancer cells love. It allows them to proliferate with little resistance from the body because the natural defense system is greatly hampered in its anti-cancer ability. Clearly, anything that augments the stressful release of cortisol will also enhance the growth of the cancer, and vice versa.

That's where meditation comes into play. Through a variety of actions and responses mediated within the autonomic nervous system, meditation diametrically opposes the fight-or-flight reaction of acute stress and reverses the insidious results of prolonged stress. The reduction of cortisol levels is one of its modes of action, certainly the most important in the reversal of the cancer process.

Another important physical result of meditation is the reduction of lactate in the blood. From measurements obtained by Robert Keith Wallace and Herbert Benson, as reported in *Scientific American*, blood lactate levels dropped precipitously in subjects who were actively meditating. During the first ten minutes of meditation, reduction in the blood lactate level occurred four times faster than in subjects who were simply resting in a reclined position. Upon cessation of the meditation, the blood lactate level continued to fall another 10 percent to reach an average of 7.3 milligrams per hundred compared to premeditation levels of 11.4 milligrams per hundred—an astonishing 30 percent drop.

Whatever the reason for this highly significant reduction in blood lactate levels, it has positive implications, both pyschological and physical, in the treatment of anxiety-related illnesses. For example, artificially increasing lactate levels in patients who suffer from anxiety neurosis bring on an acute attack. Anxiety also occurs in many healthy people who are given lactate through intravenous injection. It's no wonder, then, that meditators suffer less anxiety neurosis and less high blood pressure, another ailment commonly associated with high lactate levels.

Doctors now realize that one of the negative components of cancer is the tension and anxiety associated with the illness. The diagnosis itself is stressful, and stress is one of the contributors to the development of the condition. Thus a vicious circle arises, to the detriment of the patient. The circle must be broken.

The continued practice of meditation reduces lactate levels, with a consequential reduction in stress and anxiety. Now the patient is mentally free to rationally confront the formidable foe. With the immune system also augmented by freedom from the restraints of elevated cortisol levels, the patient has a much better chance of overcoming the problem and putting the cancer into remission. This job is also aided by the release of healing substances from the mental pharmacy.

During periods of meditation, the patterns of electrical activity in the brain are greatly modified, as amply demonstrated in 1966 by two Japanese psychiatrists, Drs. Hirai and Kasamatsu. These researchers produced the most thorough study of brain wave activity in meditating subjects. They found that during periods of meditation, the normal wakeful pattern shifts to a pattern predominated by the alpha wave activity normally recorded in profoundly relaxed and therapeutic states. Alpha is a very slow, undulating, low-frequency brain wave pattern normally present when you are at ease or "tuned into" what you are doing. Alpha activity persisted in the most artful meditators even when strong external stimuli were employed to disrupt the meditation. These meditators were able to maintain alpha activity with their eyes open—a difficult feat. There were no similarities between the brain wave patterns of meditation and either sleep or hypnosis, indicating that the state of meditation is unique unto itself.

These results show that meditation has a profound and matchless effect on the brain, an effect associated with a state of deep relaxation. But more than this, it is an effect that aids in or causes the release of the positive chemicals of good health from the brain.

We know that during periods of extreme physical exertion, such as long-distance running, the chemicals of health, the endorphins and the enkephalins, provide the added strength and will to carry on. We have seen how these substances are released during childbirth and during heroic feats so that the body can perform its function in the face of tremendous pain or adversity. And we have noted the phenomenal effects these substances can have on the natural defense system. Of the chemicals manufactured and released from the brain, they are the most powerful found to date. And evidence suggests that they are released during meditation.

Based on the overall effect of meditation on the body and the mental disposition of meditators, it seems that endorphin release may be an important part of the process. These substances are associated with joy and happiness. According to meditators, periods of intense meditation are followed by overwhelming feelings of joy and contentment. The meditators are at peace with themselves and their surroundings. They are in total harmony with life. Could these feelings be the emotional manifestation of endorphin release? Researchers think so.

The unique pattern of brain wave activity that arises during periods of meditation might also arise during the relaxation between delivery contractions or at the times a runner fades into the deep recesses of the mind, transported by the cadence of the pace and the rhythm of breathing—in fact, meditators actually use controlled breathing patterns to achieve their desired state. This whole practice of mentally stimulating the immune system is opening up quickly and promises to be one of the most exciting fields of medicine. We will soon understand the relationships between meditation and good health, but for now we can only theorize about the correlations. Regardless, the results are real.

Meditation has a proven, positive effect on the immune system. Whether this effect is solely the result of decreased cortisol release or a combination of many things—including the manufacture and release of endorphins and enkephalins from the brain, the augmentation of interferon and interleukin in the blood, or the distribution of substances yet to be discovered—it is up to you to use this powerful tool to the best of your ability. It is your personal responsibility to do whatever possible to better your chances of survival in the war against cancer and meditation is a wonderful approach with potent possibilities.

INTRODUCTION TO MEDITATION

To simplify this introduction to the practice of meditation, this chapter provides only a short description of one technique. From this presentation, you can acquire some idea of the nature of the exercise. If the concept and practice appeal to you, you will need to seek out further assistance. Since meditation is something that must be learned and practiced, you must obtain a personal instructor, someone who will work with you and provide specific techniques that will aid in your progress and appreciation.

Only after serious consideration should you attempt to use meditation as an adjunct therapy. You must be able to relate to the exercise and the experience for it to be beneficial, and you must dedicate yourself to its routine practice. Without a total acceptance and commitment on your part, the value of the meditation will be greatly limited, and the benefit will be minimal. In fact, if you were to sit down right now and attempt to meditate after reading this chapter, you would probably think there is nothing to it because nothing special happened to you. But don't be discouraged so easily. Only after weeks, perhaps even months, of active meditation, will you begin to perceive the quality of the experience. Then and only then, if you truly identify with the practice and become entrenched in the feeling and philosophy, will you realize a reward far beyond your expectations. Otherwise, the most you will experience is the reduction of stress that normally comes with meditation. This in itself is very positive, but it is not the ultimate goal of meditation.

That ultimate goal is a true self-realization—a real

understanding of yourself and the purpose of your existence. With this knowledge, you will look at life a little differently. You will reach a stage where your cancer seems unimportant compared to the other aspects of your life. You will literally transcend the pain and suffering, the negative elements of the physical world, and move to a higher plane of thought and consciousness. You will create the internal energy and the environment to make tremendous changes in yourself and your life and to dramatically affect the course of your illness.

Remember, to accomplish these results requires commitment and practice. It requires the use of proper instruction and, above all, much dedication. With these thoughts in mind, consider the practice as it is presented here.

MEDITATION EXERCISE FOR THE BEGINNER

Initially, you must find a quiet place that is free from distractions. Sit peacefully for a few minutes, then assume an appropriate posture for meditating. Generally this is a sitting position with the back straight, which means drawn in modestly at the waist and pushed out slightly in the lower back. Your weight should be evenly distributed and supported by your lower back. You should be completely comfortable.

In the proper position, your head should be in line with your hips, your ears in line with your shoulders, and your nose in line with your navel. This posture allows the correct flow of energy up and down the spine. Making minor adjustments by swaying in small circles will settle you in just the right pose, so that all of your weight drops directly down your spine.

Allow your hands to rest comfortably in your lap. Do not clasp them together rigidly, but they may touch. You can also rest them on your thighs or knees with

humbs and palms pointed upward and fingers slightly
)ent.

If you are sitting on the floor, your legs should be
)laced in the yoga position with legs crossed and feet
'esting on top of your thighs. Since this position is diffi-
:ult for most initiates, the alternative of crossing the
egs with feet resting on the floor is perfectly accept-
ıble. Another fine alternative is to sit on the front half
)f a chair with your legs extended straight in front of
'ou and your feet planted on the floor. Or, in a larger
:hair, you may sit fully to the rear of the chair and cross
'our legs as desired on the seat of the chair. The objec-
.ive is to maintain a straight posture in a comfortable
)osition.

Next, take a couple of slow, deep breaths. Breathe
:hrough your nose, not your mouth. Clear all your air
)assages, and continue to breathe completely naturally,
1ot too slowly or too rapidly, but at a pace that is regular and satisfying. Close your eyes.

Now, try not to think about anything. Just repeat to
yourself a mantra that you find appealing. A mantra is
ı word or series of words that have no concrete meaning
to the meditator. They are simply used to focus the attention away from all distractions and allow the flow of
consciousness that is the essence of meditation. A universal mantra that can be use is "ham so," the natural
sound made by the flow of air through the trachea. It is
the natural mantra of the Siddha Yoga Foundation and
is acceptable for universal applications.

Continue to repeat the mantra as you breathe, regu-
lating the words with your breath and the movement of
your chest, "ham" on the inhalation and "so" on the expi-
ration. "Ham so . . .ham so . . . ham so." Think of nothing, just repeat the mantra, and allow the flow of
thoughts that arise from deep within. Don't try to edit
those thoughts. Don't suppress them or encourage
them; just let them flow. Continue to repeat the mantra

whenever you find yourself going astray or when you become captive of a specific thought or concept. Always allow the play of consciousness to unfold in front of you and concentrate on that task; in other words, become the witness of your own mind. Focus on the origin of your inner thoughts, not the thoughts themselves. Bring your mind to a complete stop, and appreciate only your self.

As Muktanada expressed in his book *Meditate*, "Within us are infinite miracles and infinite wonders. As we go deeper into meditation, we come to understand the reality of all the different worlds we read about. Within these inner spaces, beautiful music resounds. Within us are such delicious nectars that nothing in this world can compare to them in sweetness, and there are suns so effulgent that the outer sun looks dull beside them. We should meditate systematically and with great persistence and go deeper and deeper within the body. In this way, meditation will be a gradual unfolding of our inner being." You will unfold the inner being that heals.

When the meditation period is over, you should begin to consciously refocus your attention to your surroundings. You can now open your eyes, but before you arise, quietly rest for a moment and reflect on the meditation. Recall and record the experiences that occurred in order to fully appreciate their significance. Sit momentarily and enjoy the peace and bliss that you feel, then get up and slowly resume your normal activities.

The use of meditation as an adjunct therapy requires training and practice, commitment and persistence. But this is true of all of the adjunct therapies. You must meditate several times a day for at least fifteen minutes. And you must do it religiously, without missing a few days here or a week or two there.

Some people will say that they cannot fit the activity into their busy daily schedules, that they already have too much to do and have room for nothing more. This attitude must be replaced with a concerted effort to make time or to use your time more wisely. The resultant rearrangement of commitments and priorities will help ensure the success of the meditation and also the therapy.

Although the practice of meditation appears to be a simple procedure, it can have dramatic repercussions, as our case studies have shown. It changes the internal chemistry of the body and causes the release of the substances that heal. It has a beneficial neurophysiological effect in that it breaks the vicious cycle that turns stress to cancer, cancer to stress. But beyond this, it cultivates inner reflection and awareness. It establishes a vantage point from which the patient can observe his or her interactions with the self and others, with the inner and outer world. It frequently leads to positive changes in life, modifications of lifestyle, and dramatic reversals of physical illness. This is the phenomemon of meditation. This is the phenomenon of spontaneous remission.

Recommended Reading

Brown, B. *New Mind, New Body.* New York: Harper and Row, 1975.

Muktananda. *I Am That.* South Fallsburg, NY: Siddha Yoga Dham Association, 1978.

———. *Meditate.* Albany, NY: State University of New York, 1980.

———. *Play of Consciousness.* San Francisco, CA: Harper and Row, 1978.

Pelletier, K. R. *Mind As Healer, Mind as Slayer.* New York: Dell, 1977.

Shasta Abbey. *Zen Meditation.* Mount Shasta, CA: Shasta Abbey Publications.

As an aid to both meditation and visualization, crystals have slowly made their way into the hands of metaphysical healers and those wishing to be healed. Although their effectiveness is unproven, numerous accounts have currently reached the media, accounts that include the testimonials of a wide range of people who claim to have benefited from these natural healing stones.

According to the users, each stone has a natural vibration that transmits healing energy into the area of concern. Although this is probably true, it is impossible to say whether or not this energy has curative powers. Rather, the crystals appear to allow the users themselves to focus singular attention on a troublesome area of the body and thus direct internal healing. Apparently a type of visualization or meditation is the driving force behind the cure, and the crystals become a means of channeling that healing energy.

Like so many other forms of unusual cures or therapies, the use of crystals cannot be explained. As healing objects they have their value, but they should not be placed in the class of therapies that include visualization, meditation, macrobiotics, and the others that are discussed in this book—therapies that have been scientifically shown to have tremendous value to the cancer patient. If you have a particular affinity to objects like crystals and would like to apply their mystical powers, by all means use them. But these forms of therapy are among the most unorthodox and unproven and should only be used as aids, not adjuncts.

MEDITATION CENTERS
Nationwide Programs

Himalayan Institute of
Yoga Science and
Philosophy
Centers all over United
States
Call 212-243-5994 for
information

National Yoga Teachers'
Directory
Yoga Journal, Issue No. 33
July-August 1980

The School of Tai Chi
Chuan
Centers all over United
States and Mexico
Call 212-929-1981 for
information

Siddha Yoga Dham
Association (SYDA)
South Falsburg, NY
914-434-4850

Sivananda Yoga Vedanta
Center

Centers all over United
States, Canada, and
Europe
Call 212-255-4560 for
information

Sri Chinmoy Centre
Centers in New York,
Boston, Chicago, Rhode
Island, Phoenix,
Washington and San
Francisco
Call 212- 523-3471 for
information

3HO Foundation
Centers all over United
States
Call 213-553-5662 for
information

Transcendental Meditation
Centers all over United
States, Canada, Europe,
and most college
campuses
Consult Yellow Pages

Local Centers

Academy of Taoist Arts
2750 Dwight Way #19
Berkeley, CA 94704
415-843-7580

American Buddhist
Assocation
3070 Albany Crescent
Bronx, NY 10463

American Institute for
Buddhist Studies
86 College Street
Amherst, MA 01002
413-256-0281

Ananda Ashram
Tantric Yoga
Road 3, Box 141
Monroe, NY 10950
914-782-5575

Ananda Yoga Teacher
  Training Course
Department E W
900 Allegheny Star Route
Nevada City, CA 95959

The A.R.E. Clinic
4018 North 40 Street
Phoenix, AZ 85018
602-856-6950

Association for Research
  and Enlightenment
100 Cooper Street
New York, NY 10034
212-942-1186

Buddhist Meditation
  Center
498 West End Avenue, 1-C
New York, NY 10024
212-580-9282

Center for Higher
  Consciousness
631 University Avenue,
  NE
Minneapolis, MN 55413
612-379-2386

Center for Jewish
  Meditation and Healing
15 Park Avenue
New York, NY 10016

The Center of the Light
P.O. Box 540 A
Great Barrington, MA
  01230
413-229-2396

Ch'an Meditation Center
90-31 Corona Avenue
Elmhurst, NY 11373

Chidvilas Rajneesh
  Meditation Center
154 Valley Road
Montclair, NJ 07042
201-746-9660

Chogye International Zen
  Center
39 East 31st Street
New York, NY 10016
212-683-5049

Dharmadhatu
49 East 21st Street
New York, NY 10010
212-673-7340

East West Academy of
  Healing Arts
P.O. Box 31211
San Francisco, CA 94131
415-285-9400

Foundation for Human
  Understanding
8780 Venice Boulevard
P.O. Box 34036
Los Angeles, CA 90034

Himalayan Institute
78 Fifth Avenue
New York, NY 10011
212-243-5994, 212-243-5995

Himalayan International
  Institute of Science and
  Philosophy
RD 1, Box 88
Honesdale, PA 18431

The Holistic Center of
  Pittsburgh
304 South Bouquet Street
Pittsburgh, PA 15213
412-682-7745

Interface
230 Central Street
Newton, MA 02158
617-964-7140

Jain Meditation
  International Center
120 East 86th Street
New York, NY 10028
212-722-7474

Jetsun Sakya Center
623 West 129 Street
New York, NY 10016
212-222-8683

Kalu Rinpoche Retreat
35 West 19th Street
New York, NY 10011
212-989-5989
914-297-2500
*Centers in Upstate New
York, Boston, and Montreal*

Koinonia
1400 Greenspring Valley
  Road
Stevenson, MD 21153
301-486-6262

Kripalu Center for Holistic
  Health
P.O. Box 793
Lenox, MA 01240
413-637-3234

Kundalini Research
  Foundation
475 Fifth Avenue
New York, NY 10017
212-889-3241

The Kushi Institute
E W 5 Box 110
Brookline, MA 02147
617-731-0564

The Light of Yoga Society
2134 Lee Road
Cleveland Heights, OH
  44118
216-371-0078

Meditation and Mental
  Development Center of
  New York
400 East 59th Street
New York, NY 10022
212-755-4363

Meditation Support Group
1342 B, 11 Avenue
San Francisco, CA 94122
415-566-4509

Monroe Institute of
  Applied Sciences
P.O. Box 57
Afton, VA 22920

Nataraja Yoga Ashram
3033 Central Avenue
San Diego, CA 92105
714-282-2111

Nyingmapa School of
  Tibetan Buddhism
19 West 16th Street
New York, NY 10011
212-691-8523

The Rudrananda Ashram
  (Kundalini Yoga)
519 Broadway
New York, NY 10012
212-966-6473

The School of Tai Chi
  Chuan
412 Sixth Avenue, 5th
  Floor
New York, NY 10011
212-543-5530

Sivananda Yoga Vedanta
Center
243 West 24th Street
New York, NY 10011

Sri Chinmoy Centers
765 United Nations Plaza,
Suite 2D
New York, NY 10017

Student International
Meditation Society
113 East 58th Street
New York, NY 10022
212-826-6620

Sufi Order
Box 587
Lebanon Springs, NY
12114
518-794-8080

S Y D A Foundation
324 West 86th Street
New York, NY 10024
212-724-3925

3HO Foundation
P.O. Box 35006
Los Angeles, CA 90036
213-553-5662

The Tibet Center
114 East 28th Street
New York, NY 10016
212-684-8245

University of Oriental
Studies
939 South New Hampshire
Avenue
Los Angeles, CA 90006
213-487-1235, 213-384-0850

University of the Trees
P.O. Box 644
13165 Pine Street
Boulder Creek, CA 95006

World Yoga Center
265 West 72nd Street
New York, NY 10023
212-787-4908

Wu Mei Kung Fu
307-309 Canal Street
New York, NY 10013
212-966-5063

Yoga and Growth Center of
Bergen County
84 East Ridgewood Avenue
Ridgewood, NJ 07450
201-447-2474

Yogi Gupta New York
Centre
112 Central Park South
#510
New York, NY 10019
212-247-1681

The Yoga Institute
2168 Portsmouth Street
Houston, TX 77098
713-526-6674

Yoga Meditation Study
Group
Route #1
Woodbury, TN 37190

Yoga Research Foundation
6111 SW 74 Avenue
Miami, FL 33143
305-595-5580

Zen Arts Center
P.O. Box 197
Mount Tremper, NY 12457
914-688-2228

The Zen Studies Society
New York Zendo
233 East 67th Street
New York, NY 10021

Meditation Centers of S Y D A

Siddha Yoga
1004 SW First Avenue
Gainesville, FL 32601
904-375-7629

Siddha Yoga Dham
1520 Hill
Ann Arbor, MI 48104
313-994-5625

Siddha Yoga Dham
Fernwood Road, Manor
 House
Chestnut Hill, MA 02167
617-734-0137

Siddha Yoga Dham
P.O. Box 10191
Honolulu, HI 96816
808-732-1558

Siddha Yoga Dham
3815 Garott
Houston, TX 77006
713-529-0006

Siddha Yoga Dham
605 South Mariposa
Los Angeles, CA 90005
213-386-2328

Siddha Yoga Dham
P.O. Box 52-3464
Miami, FL 33152
305-261-8924

Siddha Yoga Dham
P.O. Box 11071
Oakland, CA 94611
415-655-8677

Siddha Yoga Dham
6429 Wayne Avenue
Philadelphia, PA 19119
215-849-0888

Siddha Yoga Dham
1409 NE 66th
Seattle, WA 98115
206-523-2853

Siddha Yoga Dham
1834 Swann Street, NW
Washington, DC 20009
202-667-0842

Siddha Yoga Meditation
 Ashram
2100 West Bradley Place
Chicago, IL 60618
312-327-0536

Meditation Centers of Himalayan Institute

Amar Studio
6504 80th Street
Cabin John, MD 20818

Center for Health
 Enhancement
Professional Plaza
723 South State Street
Clarks Summit, PA 18411

Center for Higher
 Consciousness
631 University Avenue,
 NE
Minneapolis, MN 55413

Himalayan Institute at
 East West Books
78 Fifth Avenue
New York, NY 10011

Himalayan Institute
Chicago South
9703 South Forest
Chicago, IL 60628

Himalayan Institute of
Buffalo
871 Delaware Avenue
Buffalo, NY 14209

Himalayan Institute of
Dallas/Ft. Worth
3833 Diamond Loch West
Ft. Worth, TX 76118

Himalayan Institute of
Germany
Am Alten Markt 12 a
2070 Ahrensburg
West Germany

Himalayan Institute of
Glenview
1505 Greenwood Road
Glenview, IL 60025

Himalayan Institute of
India
710 Sarvapriya Bihar,
New Delhi, India

Himalayan Institute of
Indianapolis
2370 East 52nd Street
Indianapolis, IN 46205

Himalayan Institute of
Milwaukee
3581 South Kinnickinnic
Avenue
Milwaukee, WI 53207

Himalayan Institute of
Pittsburgh
5604 Solway Street,
Room 306
Pittsburgh, PA 15217

Lotus Yoga Center
109 South Roselle Road
Schaumburg, IL 60193

New Age Center for
Health Enhancement
122 Speedwell Avenue
Morristown, NJ 07960

The Toronto Group
c/o 359 Sackville Street
Toronto, ON Canada M5A
3G4

The Yoga Center
1710 Houston Street
Austin, TX 78756

Yoga—Meditation Center
4232 Highview Place
Minnetonka, MN 55345

Yoga Society of Madison
320 State Street
Madison, WI 53703

11
Visualization and the Remission of Cancer

Five in one hundred were the best odds the doctors could offer a sixty-one-year-old man who in 1971 entered a hospital of the University of Oregon medical school with weakness, extreme weight loss, difficulty swallowing, and troubled breathing. His disease had progressed to the point that he could hardly swallow his own saliva, let alone solid food. And the devastating result, a drop in weight to 98 pounds, had left him too weak to function. Unfortunately, he would probably never get to see his sixty-second birthday. Instead, he would most likely die from the carcinoma that resided in his throat.

In cases such as this, it is sometimes better to withhold therapy rather than put the patient through unnecessary pain and suffering with little chance of significant improvement. Many times the patient personally confronts this dilemma and is asked to make the final decision alone. But in this particular instance, the doctors decided for him and attempted to mount a last-ditch effort in his behalf. This time the effort paid off.

The patient was prescribed a course of radiation therapy in the hope that his tumor would at least shrink and thereby allow the ingestion of solid food. A total cure was not at all expected because of the advanced stage of the illness, but a reduction in the size of the tumor was hoped for. That would provide the outside possibility of some degree of life extension, be it weeks, months, or maybe a year. The chances were slim indeed, but hope was not abandoned. Therapy was begun.

In addition to the radiation, a completely new form of therapy was employed in this case. The patient was instructed to visualize the process by which the tumor cells were being destroyed. He was asked to view the radiation as millions of miniature bullets, striking and killing all malignant cells in their path, zapping the weaker, more vulnerable parasites in preference to the surrounding normal, healthy cells that were much stronger and able to handle the devastating radiation.

Far more important than this, the patient was requested to visualize the ultimate means of tumor cell annihilation—the complete battle between the malignant enemy and the body's natural defense against cancer. He was told how his white blood cells would converge on and consume the dying or dead tumor cells, how they would carry the defeated enemy from the internal battleground to the everwaiting liver and kidneys, where the remnants of the once-threatening foe would be flushed from the body forever. He was told to visualize a gradual reduction in the size of the tumor and his return to full health when the cancer had been completely eliminated. He was told to envision health in place of illness, life instead of death.

What happened next was completely beyond the expectations or even the imagination of the attending physicians. Certainly they had all seen improvement in terminal cancer patients, but nothing quite like this. The radiation treatments were working much better than anticipated and with hardly any deleterious side effects to the normal tissue of the mouth and throat. The tumor was shrinking so rapidly that midway through the therapy, the patient once again was able to eat. Slowly but steadily, he began to regain his strength and weight as his cancer progressively vanished before the eyes of his hospital physicians. Within two more months, he showed absolutely no signs of any cancer and had reentered society a new man with a new skill.

Since the visualization had worked so well on the cancer, the man decided to attempt to relieve his arthritis through the same technique. He pictured the white blood cells of his body first preparing, then repaving the surfaces of the joints of his arms and legs. He imagined them carrying away all the debris of previous inflammations, patching any defects, leaving the joints shiny and slippery smooth. He envisioned the youthful, healthy condition that had existed before the attacks. Sure enough, he restored the joints to good function, and, like the cancer, the arthritis slowly resolved.

Next this man revamped his sex life. Unable to have intercourse for twenty years because of impotence, he applied the visualization therapy to improving his sexual potency. Within a few weeks, he was restored to full sexual activity. Here was yet another overwhelming example of his ability to willfully influence his physical health through mental imagery.

The case as presented here is completely documented and portrayed faithfully and accurately. It comes from the annals of O. Carl Simonton and appears in a more complete form in his book *Getting Well Again*, a highly recommended guide to visualization therapy and an excellent source of information on stress and cancer. Other cases and examples of successful visualization have been recorded by numerous other doctors and researchers, notably Jeanne Achterberg in her book *Imagery in Healing*; Elmer Green, Alyce Green, and Patricia A. Norris at the Menninger Foundation; Larry LeShan in his years of clinical work in New York; J. H. Schultz in the study entitled "Autogenic Training;" plus many others including the French gynecologist Fernand Lamaze of the Lamaze childbirth fame and Michael Samuels in his terrific books *Be Well, Seeing With the Mind's Eye*, and *The Well Body Book*.

RELAXATION AND MENTAL IMAGERY

Relaxation and mental imagery, as they apply to physical healing, are intended to put the participant back in touch with his or her feelings, sensations, and bodily perceptions. The two techniques help to provide an understanding of the workings of the mind-body connection and the influence of beliefs, both positive and negative, on physical and mental health. Mental imagery can be used to create positive beliefs that ultimately lead to positive health. But before you can initiate the technique of visualization, you must achieve true relaxation of the mind and body.

One of the principle functions of relaxation exercises is to put the mind and body at ease. This is accomplished through the elimination of stress so that a state of deep internal relaxation extends from the conscious mind to the physical body. Breathing becomes slower and deeper, the heart rate subsides, and the muscles of the body release their tension. Associated with all of these events is a change in wave rhythms in the brain, proving once again that the mind can have a direct effect on involuntary physical functions.

In terms of attacking cancer, the relaxation has a further benefit; it reduces the tension that is associated with the diagnosis of malignancy. If you are a cancer patient, you need not be reminded of the internal anguish that arose when you were given the shocking news that you have cancer. If you are not a cancer patient, consider your likely response to the diagnosis: feelings of anger, frustration, and remorse; fear of the pain and suffering; the thought of death itself. Compound these reflections with family and financial concerns, and you have buckets brimming with worry.

This is why relaxation procedures are so important to the cancer patient. They greatly help to eliminate the intense feelings that parallel the disease and provide a more peaceful mental and physical environment that allows healing messages to arise from the inner self. These messages change the perception of the patient so that the illness and the circumstances surrounding it can go to work for, instead of against, him or her. With a clear and relaxed mind, the patient can reflect on past and future events. A true communion with one's self can transpire, and a precise plan for dealing with life's problems can take shape. The patient is placed in a position from which to direct the course of not only the illness but life events as well. Now add the process of mental imagery, and you have the setting for some remarkable happenings, including the remission of cancer.

It is important to note that relaxation as it is discussed here does not refer to the easygoing activities associated with recreation, rest, and recuperation. Therapeutic relaxation does not mean sipping a glass of white wine and watching the afternoon soaps or popping a frosty beer and viewing the evening ball game. While these are certainly not stressful activities, neither are they associated with the deep relaxation response that leads to real stress reduction and the preparation for healing. True therapeutic relaxation is a state of mind and body achieved through the use of specific techniques that relieve tension and stress. Real relaxation is the first step in breaking that horrible negative loop of ill feelings generating illness generating ill feelings. Deep relaxation is therapeutic in the true sense of the word.

Here's one of many techniques that produces the desired state. First, before attempting relaxation, seclude yourself from all surrounding distractions—no telephone, no television, no radio, nothing but you and your consciousness. You must make an absolute commitment to dedicate five to ten minutes of your undivided time to achieve a state of relaxation that sets the stage for the practice of visualization. When you are ready, you can employ the following guidelines to assist you in your quest for complete inner peace and tranquility:

1. Find a quiet place with soft lighting and comfortable seating.

2. Make yourself cozy, either sitting or lying down. Close your eyes.

3. Concentrate on your breathing, taking several slow deep inspirations and soft prolonged expirations.

4. Concentrate on your face. Isolate and dissolve away any tension that you feel. Notice how the relaxation spreads to other parts of your body.

5. Move your thoughts to the muscles of your neck, and relax them. Next, your shoulders. Then your arms. Continue this way until you have successfully melted away the tension of your entire body.

6. Always return to your breathing if you lose concentration. Focus on the slow movement of air in and out of the lungs, the movement of the chest and the abdomen, the subtle sound of respiration.

7. When you have relaxed your entire body, remain quietly in the same location and position for a few minutes. Continue to concentrate on your slow, steady breathing.

8. After the few minutes pass, slowly open your eyes and readjust to your surroundings.

9. Now you are ready to resume normal activities or engage in mental imagery. The entire process should take 10–15 minutes.

This series of steps represents just one technique of achieving a state of relaxation; several others can be used. If you elect to practice mental imagery as an adjunct therapy, study other methods of relaxation and choose the one best suited to your nature. Regardless of which method you choose, you must arrive at the same desired goal of stress elimination, which prepares you for a session of mental imagery.

THE VISUALIZATION PROCESS

The next step is the actual process of visualization—mentally altering expectations of future events by forming an image of what is desired. For example, in Olympic high-diving competition, the participants are taught to visualize their dives before they actually perform them. By forming a mental image of the perfect plunge, the athlete psychically programs his or her body to duplicate the picture seen by the mind's eye. The result: dives that are better and scores that are higher. Likewise, golfers visualize their shots before they swing their clubs, and dancers mentally perform their routines before ever entering the stage. Extensive psychological testing has shown the value of mental imagery techniques in all fields of activity, and experts have extended its use to cancer therapy.

Like the patient in the case study at the beginning of this chapter, you can learn to use visualization to destroy and eliminate cancer or any other disease that strikes you. Even if you are not ill, you can use mental imagery to maintain well-being and good health. The technique is universal; the application is individual.

For cancer patients, the technique will most certainly be life-extending and possibly life-saving. Visualizing the destruction of a tumor directs the internal forces of natural defense and greatly enhances their effectiveness. With positive, powerful images, the mind sends concrete messages to the body, messages that command tumor cell annihilation and the restoration of good health.

The visualization can be realistic. You can view tumor cells and white blood cells in their natural forms, imagining their struggle as it actually occurs within the body. Or you can picture the entire scene symbolically, with tumor cells portrayed as tiny, scared fish schooled in a group that lacks direction, and white blood cells as fierce white sharks attacking with big teeth and ferocious appetites, devouring and digesting their timid prey. Other forms abound. The tumor cells can be visualized as frightened mice and blood cells as hungry hawks. Or use snakes and wolves, frogs and alligators. The examples are endless, and the choice is up to you. In any case, envision the cancer as the weaker form and the blood cells as the stronger, victorious opponents.

According to Jeanne Achterberg and supported by the research of other scientists and therapists, the characteristics of the images go far to predict the outcome of the therapy. For example, when asked to imagine the color of their tumors, patients described a host of colors from yellow to black. It was later determined that the softer colors of blue and green were associated with less intense feelings about the cancer and a poorer prognosis, whereas the colors of red and black evoked stronger convictions that led to more positive antitumor action. These results were recorded by R. L. Trestman of the University of Tennessee in Knoxville.

Furthermore, when patients viewed the elements of the natural defense system in vague or conflicting terms, the course of the therapy was less than desirable.

White blood cells represented by snowflakes or clouds connoted a weak image of the immune system and also a frail image of self. How could these imaginary warriors ever destroy a malignant enemy? White blood cells represented by wolves and sharks, certainly more powerful forms, were linked with positive therapeutic results, but they were not the best images to associate with the cells of the immune system. The best forms, according to Achterberg, were "archetypal figures who fought for God and country and who were protectors of the people, such as Sir Richard or the knights of the Round Table. These images are not only powerful, they are also pure, righteous champions of good and just causes.

When the cancer was viewed as strong, overpowering, or irrepressible, a poor outcome was predicted. Cancer images like coal, crabs, or insects were almost impossible to overcome and consequently not well controlled, destroyed, or eliminated. Patients dealt with weaker cancer forms, like helpless, timid animals or soft mutable objects, in a more positive fashion and achieved much better results.

Still another component is generally added to the mental drama—the therapeutic agent being received by the patient. Chemotherapy is seen as poison that further weakens the tumor cells but not the white blood cells; radiation is seen as tiny bullets or laser beams that also aid in the destruction of the cancer. Again, it's up to the patient to decide exactly what images make the most sense or which ones are the easiest to conceive, and then to form a mental picture and act out the scenario.

As an example, consider the following scene, and mentally visualize the good characters performing their life-saving functions. Think of the cancer as fragile and helpless. Think of the white blood cell characters as strong and noble, fighting for your survival. Then envision the drama that will end in the destruction and elimination of the cancer through the efforts of your natural defenses.

Example #1:

VISUALIZED IMAGE #1

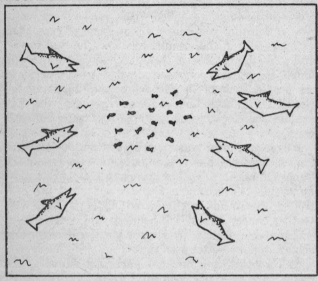

This example is a forceful image. The chemotherapeutic liquid ⌒ has drugged and weakened the tiny helpless bait fish, ⊂⇒ the tumor cells, making them even more vulnerable for the great white sharks ⊂⇒ (the white blood cells). Imagine the attack of the sharks as they converge on the helpless fish and devour every one of them, digesting the remains of their engulfed bodies until nothing is left.

Now think back on the function of white blood cells and the process of phagocytosis as described in Chapter 3, "What You Need to Know About Cancer." Remember how macrophages engulf and digest their natural enemies: bacteria, viruses, and cancer cells. This is the process you should envision in your mental dramas between imaginary characters of good and evil, the white blood cell sharks and the tiny, fragile, malignant bait fish.

Example #2:

VISUALIZED IMAGE #2

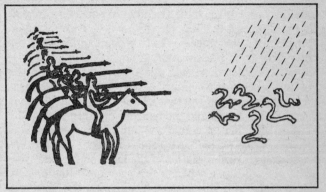

This second image is more powerful than the first. In addition to a strong portrayal of the white blood cell images and a weak representation of the cancer images, there is also the association of good and evil in the two sets of characters. The knights in shining armor are protected from the falling rain of chemotherapeutic drugs, chemicals that poison the cancerous enemy. The knights represent a force of goodness that is ready to overcome the evil group of weak and confused snakes.

Now play out this drama in your own mind. Consider the conclusion. The gallant knights gather all the helpless evil snakes and systematically destroy them all until the kingdom is once again safe, purged of all the forces that bring illness and destruction to the realm. In like manner, the forces of the GOOD SYSTEM of the body contain and destroy the tumor cells to which they are directed by the mind.

The process of visualization should be controlled by therapists who have appropriate training. Under their instruction, the patient is encouraged to assume a comfortable position, generally a reclining pose, and listen to a relaxation message provided by the therapist or a tape recording. Following this message, the therapists suggest a brief description of the disease process (how the tumor came into being) and the healing process (how the natural defense system of the body will eliminate the tumor). You have already learned this information in Chapters 3 and 4. Use it to increase your understanding of both processes so that you can increase the potency of your visualization.

The therapist then asks the patient to imagine the healing process at work, just as you were asked to visualize the outcome of the two different symbolic dramas between the sharks and the fish and the knights and the animals. During an actual session, no specific scene is drawn for the patient. All representations are left entirely up to the imagination of the listener, but the therapist may question what the cancer looks like or how the immune cells will destroy it. The intention is only to guide the patient in the right direction and stimulate thoughts that will assist in the creation of positive images. The exact characters the patient envisions will mirror the patient's feelings about the illness and him or herself. The visualization script the patient acts out will reflect his or her understanding of the healing process and the patient's ability to control it. These aspects of the visualization process will determine the effectiveness of the treatment and are best left to the patient's imagination.

A YOUNG PATIENT

Unless the individual creates personally meaningful characters, the entire exercise may be useless, and the patient may become frustrated by the experience. It is only through a strong association and relationship with the good forces of the natural defense system that the patient will be able to project him or herself into the struggle. To appreciate the value of the patient's input in the visualization script, consider a case study from the Menninger Foundation as discussed by Patricia Norris in one of the foundation's publications.

In this case, the patient was a nine-year-old boy who awoke one morning with a numbness in his left arm. Initially, this insensitivity was dismissed as nothing more than discomfort caused by sleeping in the wrong position. But the symptom persisted, and one day the child awoke with complete paralysis of his arm and was taken for immediate medical care.

His doctors didn't take long to diagnose the problem. With the aid of a CAT scan, a specialized three-dimensional form of x-ray, they determined that the young boy harbored a malignant tumor within the right side of his brain. Inoperable by virtue of its size and placement, the astrocytoma was composed of brain cells that had somehow gone wild and grown unrestricted, displacing normal brain tissue and compressing the vital area in the brain that controlled the child's arm.

Something had to be done quickly, or the tumor would continue to grow and compress additional brain tissue, producing more severe symptoms and ultimately taking the boy's life. Since the tumor was considered inoperable, instead of surgery, the child was given a full course of radiation therapy, the next best treatment for astrocytoma. He was given all that he could tolerate, and when the regimen was complete, he was sent home with the hope that the symptoms would abate.

But as time passed, the worst possibilities were realized. His symptoms did not diminish. Instead, they continued to increase in severity to involve his left leg and most of the left side of his body. Since chemotherapy is of questionable benefit in cases of astrocytoma, and no more radiation could be tolerated, his doctors said they had done all they could, that they had exhausted all traditional modes of therapy, that they had nothing else to offer.

Fortunately for the child, his parents had something

else to offer. They were aware of a revolutionary new cancer treatment, a program that involved the patient in his own therapy—a self-controlled plan to mobilize the body's natural defense system to stage an internal fight against malignancy. To assist their son in his attempt to overcome his illness, the parents obtained one of the mental imagery tapes made by the Cancer Research and Treatment Center in Fort Worth, Texas, and with the professional guidance available at the Menninger Foundation in Topeka, Kansas, the young boy was introduced to a special form of "mental" cure, a cure on which he staked his life.

After several attempts to use the relaxation and imagery tape, the child became discontented with the program and decided to make one of his own, using his own visual scenario. Since he was an avid fan of Star Trek and other space adventures, he decided to program his ego as a space squadron commander who was in charge of protecting the galaxy (his brain) from an invading alien (the tumor). His natural weapons, the white blood cells of his body, were represented by lasers and torpedoes, which constituted the arsenal controlled by the fleet of fighter planes. Mentally, he controlled those weapons; psychologically, he bombed his tumor.

In addition to this fantasy form of abstract visualization, concrete visualization was also employed, and in time this became the main component of the routine. Instead of conceptualizing rocket launchers and torpedoes, the child was instructed to envision the actual white blood cells that the imaginary weapons represented. He was taught to picture the destruction of the tumor by the ever-present and ever-hungry blood cells, and he often represented them in drawings as large balls with round mouths lined with many teeth. He saw hundreds of them attacking and eating up the tumor until nothing was left.

Also, at the onset of the imagery training, the child was taught basic techniques of biofeedback, such as

warming the hands to ninety-seven degrees, deep muscle relaxation, and maintaining very low muscular tension for extended periods of time. These techniques
were extremely important, not only to allow the child to
relax and to dissipate his anxiety, but also to demon-
strate that the mind and the body are connected. This
realization was naturally extended to the visualization.
After all, if the mind could direct warmth to the hands
and extend relaxation to the muscles, why couldn't it
direct white blood cells to the tumor and effectively
eradicate it?

Then a final component of the mental therapy was
drawn into play: the unconscious. As a final and continuing step in the treatment, the therapist at the Menninger Foundation explained to the child that what he had
envisioned during his imagery sessions was really a
process that occurred naturally. Although he was consciously directing this natural defense mechanism and
enhancing its effectiveness, it was always at work,
fighting the tumor day and night, aided by an internal
commander who was always on duty.

This subtle but powerful suggestion was of the ut-
most importance because it allowed the white blood
cells to continue their battle even when the child was
not consciously controlling them. They were directed in
their effort by an unconscious force similar to a post-
hypnotic suggestion, and continuously reinforced by
the child's own volition. But would this therapy really
be able to help the child in his fight for life, or did it
merely distract the child from feeling despair and
doom?

Immediately following the radiation treatments, the
child's condition took a turn for the worse, and his clinical picture continued to deteriorate during the first few
months of mental imagery training. Of necessity he was
put into a leg brace, which he required in order to walk,
and he needed assistance to arise whenever he fell. His
future looked bleak, so his doctors ordered a second

CAT scan in order to better determine what was actually occurring inside his head. The results were discouraging; the tumor had grown much larger.

At this point the child was facing his own mortality and began to question those around him about the possibility of imminent death. His father was truthful and did not negate the possibility but remained positive and supportive. His therapist reduced the question to a choice: Did the child choose to live or die? That was the real point.

The child chose life.

He worked harder than ever with his mental imagery and received constant encouragement from his parents and therapist. They never lost confidence in the ultimate success of the therapy, even though the odds were certainly stacked against the child. He fought the tumor with a playful spirit and a oneness of purpose until suddenly things began to turn his way.

Physically he started to improve. His leg strengthened, and he could arise without assistance whenever he fell. His arm improved, affording more use. And his overall health improved to project a much better appearance. Finally one day, he announced that he could no longer "see" the tumor. It was completely destroyed. No matter where he searched within the confines of his brain, he was unable to locate the enemy invader, the thief of life. Still he continued with his mental imagery and envisioned his white blood cells searching endlessly for any stragglers that might have escaped eradication. Although he never pictured the tumor again and had full faith that it indeed was gone, he still desired some real proof that it was totally demolished. A third CAT scan was ordered.

Although it was much delayed because the physicians thought it was unnecessary, a series of physical problems and falls that plagued the child during this period of high anticipation eventually forced the issue, and the CAT scan was ordered. After the full series was completed, the news was released. *There was no sign of the tumor anywhere.* Without any further treatments, without chemotherapy and without surgery, the tumor had been eradicated. The child was in remission.

Even though his doctors were skeptical and felt that the visualization had played no role in the cure, the young patient, his parents, and therapist all knew otherwise. They had suffered through the shortcomings of traditional treatments, observed the physical deterioration that followed the radiation therapy, and witnessed the remarkable comeback and miraculous cure that occurred with the biofeedback and visualization techniques. They rejoiced in their success.

It was the child who really understood what had happened. As he put it, the radiation softened the tumor and made it easier for him to destroy it. Be that as it may, and this is probably the closest view to the truth, it was the child who went the extra distance on his own, crossing the finish line to win the race and his life. He truly "masterminded" his own miracle by pushing the imaginary buttons of an imaginary game that took place within his brain.

Recommended Reading

Achterberg, J. *Imagery in Healing*. Boston: New Science Library, 1985.

Benson, H. *The Relaxation Response*. New York: Morrow, 1975.

LeShan, L. L. *You Can Fight for Your Life*. New York: M. Evans and Company, 1977.

Samuels, M. and H. Bennett. *The Well Body Book*. New York: Random House-Bookworks, 1973.

Samuels, M., and N. Samuels. *Seeing with the Mind's Eye*. New York: Random House-Bookworks, 1975.

Simonton, O. C., S. Simonton and J. Creighton. *Getting Well Again*. Los Angeles: Tarcher, 1978.

VISUALIZATION AND BIOFEEDBACK THERAPY CENTERS, CLINICS, AND FOUNDATIONS

Associated Biofeedback
Medical Group
71-35 110 Street
Forest Hills, NY 11375

Biofeedback Consultation
Service
310 Madison Avenue
New York, NY 10017
212-687-0180

Biofeedback Society of
New Jersey
P.O. Box 686
Franklin Park, NJ 08823

Biofeedback Society of
New York
115 East 87th Street
New York, NY 10128

Biofeedback Study Center
of New York
55 East 9th Street
New York, NY 10003
212-673-4710

Cancer Care Center
11770 East Warner Avenue
Fountain Valley, CA 92708

Cancer Counseling Center
6060 North Central
Expressway
Suite 140
Dallas, TX 75206
214-373-7744

Cancer Counseling Center
875 Via de la Paz
Suite C
Pacific Palisades, CA
90272
203-459-4434

The Menninger Foundation
Biofeedback and
Psychophysiology Center
5800 SW 6th Avenue
Topeka, KS 66606
913-273-7500
*Drs. Elmer Green and
Alyce Green have a referral
list of physicians,
psychotherapists, and
clinical psychologists
around the country who are
qualified to counsel
patients.*

Robert Price, M.D.
Simonton Method
205 West Walnut Avenue
San Diego, CA 92103
619-373-7744

Leonne Schillo, R.N., M.N.
Health Image
23300 Ventura Boulevard,
Suite 1
Woodland Hills, CA 91364
818-887-5743

Visualization Tapes
Organelle Manipulation
(OM) Corporation
Wilmette, IL 60091

12
Hypnosis and the Remission of Cancer

The mind plays an amazingly strong role in the genesis and maintenance of malignancies. From the studies of Galen, a medical observer of the second century, we learn that women who suffered severe personal losses and experienced prolonged remorse and depression were highly susceptible to the subsequent occurrence of cancer (negative mind over matter, the BAD SYSTEM at work). And for centuries, mental causes of cancer were as well established in the journals of medicine as viral and environmental causes are today.

Consider the views of Sigmund Freud, who saw cancer purely as a psychologically generated illness, a conflict between the libido and the ego. Similarly, Elida Evans in 1926 analyzed 100 cancer patients and found the great majority to exhibit basically the same type of psychological dependencies and dilemmas. These were characterized by a strong emotional dependence upon another person or a specific external object. With the loss of that object or person came the hopelessness and helplessness that contemporary researchers describe today, soon to be followed by a malignant process. In 1937 Wilhelm Reich advanced the notion that character resignation and emotional lassitude form the psychological platform from which cancer springs. Reich rationalized that weak emotional states are associated with the weak biological constitutions that ultimately lead to cellular degeneration and cancer.

Regardless of how far one wishes to carry the concept, the correlations between emotions and cancer are endless: leukemia in children who experience overwhelming sibling rivalry; lymphoma in patients recently separated from a strong parental figure; malignancies in women just widowed. Many other similar cases seem to show the power of negative mind over matter, the BAD SYSTEM at work. As Woody Allen expressed in his movie *Manhattan*, "I don't get angry, I just grow a tumor."

If a tumor is really the outward manifestation of repressed emotions, as we are led to believe by these many medical researchers and practitioners, then those emotions must be confronted and eliminated before the malignant process can be reversed. Encouragingly, numerous psychologists and psychiatrists now concur that hypnosis is a useful tool to unlock the chains that bind the mind in depression and despair, hatred and rage, thereby freeing the mental powers and then directing them to eliminate cancer.

Hypnosis, in its earliest form, is perhaps the most ancient type of treatment used to fight disease. In her book *Imagery in Healing*, Achterberg points out the healing powers of the shamans, dating back 10,000 years or more, probably account for the first "cures" that were consciously directed. Primitive shaman healers, armed only with the words they spoke and the symbols they used, effectively exorcized the demons thought to cause disease, thereby eliminating not only the symptoms but also the causes of the illness. Thousands of years later, the Chinese were to write that the highest form of healing employed no medicines or instruments whatsoever. Instead, disease was treated by the manipulation of the mind through the spoken word of the healer. A thousand years thereafter, numerous accounts in the New Testament describe the many cures generated through the speech and gestures of Jesus Christ, cures brought about completely through the power of the healing word.

More recently, in the early nineteenth century, proponents of the first form of modern hypnosis, a practice called mesmerism, claimed to have cured all sorts of illnesses, illnesses that would not respond to any of the available therapies of the day, illnesses that were both mental and physical. Today, modern hypnosis has been used effectively in the treatment of a wide variety of maladies that include high blood pressure, obesity, unrelenting neurological pain, neuroses, and even common warts.

But what about cancer? Is it really possible to affect the course of such an illness using only words and symbols? Can hypnosis have any effect on such a difficult problem, a problem that is generally viewed as purely physical, not mental? To answer these questions, consider that electric shock given to depressed cancer patients frequently causes a reduction in the malignancy. Amazingly, shocking the mind can awaken the immune system, and cancer can be reversed. On the therapeutic level, hypnosis can be used to shock the mind.

Well documented in contemporary medical literature are innumerable examples of a variety of mental ailments and physical problems that have responded well to hypnotic cures. Generally, the hypnosis was used in conjunction with other, more traditional therapies, as an aid rather than a primary choice of treatment. Nevertheless, the results have been real, greater than what normally would have been expected. Frequently too, the hypnosis was used as a last resort, when all other treatments had failed and the disease had progressed to an extremely difficult point. Under these conditions, positive results are even more impressive, and the powers of the "spoken word" are seen in full light. Still, until now, few have attempted to harness those powers to direct the mind to eliminate malignancy.

In principle, hypnosis is closely associated with the process of visualization. Both forms of therapy use the powers of the mind to direct the body's natural defenses in a positive and beneficial way, focusing the attention of the immune system and promoting the release of natural healing substances.

Hypnosis can also be used as an escape that breaks the cycle of fear, cancer, and more fear, or of depression, cancer, and more depression. It can allow the mind to relax, to let go of the problem and temporarily shift its focus to something or someone else. This escape, this temporary release, will set up the conditions for a remission. It will allow the mind to shift from the BAD SYSTEM to the GOOD SYSTEM and in so doing generate the chemicals that destroy cancer cells.

Hypnosis can work in other ways as well, for example, in combination with other therapies or as the driving force behind those therapies. Take, for instance, the case of the young boy who fought his brain tumor with self-directed visualization, as described in Chapter 11. He performed the mental imagery in a couple of sessions each day but was also instructed in a form of hypnotic suggestion to continue to fight the tumor mentally and physically, hour after hour, day after day, asleep or awake. As you will recall, his success could have been attributed to a number of different things, but most likely it was the combination of them all, including the verbal suggestion.

In combination with the standard treatments of surgery, radiation, and chemotherapy, hypnotic suggestion can increase the potency of these treatments while at the same time bolstering the power of the natural defense system. As perhaps the most powerful form of the healing word, hypnosis can be used to fill the void of purely psychologically directed cures. And since the practice has already been shown to work within the constraints of its limited use, imagine the potential in years to come when current techniques are improved. Hypnosis is definitely the cancer cure of mind over matter. It is yesterday's and tomorrow's cure that can be used today.

Introduction to Hypnosis

This basic introduction to hypnosis is intended to help you evaluate the practice and determine whether it is right for you. Hypnosis should be especially considered as an adjunct therapy if you believe your illness has a strong psychological component or if you fit into the personality types most prone to cancer.

Hypnosis is a misunderstood practice. In the past, it has been wrongly associated with magic and witchcraft, spiritualism and voodoo, although it is totally unrelated to these practices. Today it is an established technique that has been used successfully in appropriate cases by trained practitioners, mostly psychologists and psychiatrists in clinical settings. It is taught in some of the finest medical schools in this country and around the world.

The rationale behind the use of hypnosis in the treatment of cancer is the well-established fact that there is often a strong psychological basis for malignancy. Through hypnosis, this internal strife is exposed, and the patient is taught to understand his or her problems. This understanding enables the patient to initiate positive, health-giving changes in his or her thoughts, feelings, and attitudes.

Since the human mind is extremely vulnerable to suggestion, it is constantly being swayed by external stimuli or suggestive thoughts and ideas that arise from within. Most psychological suffering is the result of negative thoughts that seep from the deep recesses of our subconsciousness and flood our mind. Past experiences of guilt, denied feelings, and repressed desires float into our awareness, causing confusion and anxiety, depriving us of our happiness and our health. Over a period of many years, this negativism becomes engraved in our thinking and in our actions, persisting like a bad habit. The process of hypnosis provides the tools to break this bad habit, to replace the negative thinking with positive thoughts and ideas.

People usually have difficulty working out their emotional and psychological problems by themselves; they are too close to the problems to evaluate them properly. After all, with your nose up against the billboard, it's hard to see the whole picture. Consequently, at times it becomes necessary to seek out professional help in the resolution of psychological and emotional conflicts. This is not an indication of a weakness or the sign of mental illness, but rather an intelligent approach to a difficult dilemma. So if you think there is psychological component to your illness, don't feel embarrassed about asking for professional help from a psychiatrist or psychologist. Just remember, bad habits and negative thinking took years to develop, so don't expect overnight success in reversing the tendencies. It takes hard work, dedication, and persistence to reverse years of negative patterns, and hypnosis can definitely help.

Two questions commonly arise in the discussion of hypnosis as potential therapy. The first is whether everyone can be hypnotized. The answer is simple: yes, everyone can be hypnotized. In fact, hypnosis is a natural state that each of us experiences just before we fall asleep. In the treatment session, this state is prolonged as much as possible so that the therapist can work within its frame. Of course, it is possible to resist the hypnotic state, just as one would fight the tendency to fall asleep, but in time and with practice, the resistance can be subdued, and the hypnotic state can be induced to the full.

The second question commonly asked is what hypnosis feels like. Here the answer is more subjective, because the feeling can vary from one person to another and depends on the depth of hypnosis that is achieved. Put simply, entering the hypnotic state is similar to the feeling of just starting to fall asleep. You will remain conscious, and you will be aware of your surroundings. Your mind will be alert, and your thoughts will remain under your control. You will linger somewhere between wakefulness and sleep, nodding but not actually sleeping. This is the most desirable state, because the mind is most open to suggestion at this time. Some people will eventually fall asleep, while others remain awake throughout the entire procedure; this is irrelevant. The important thing is that you enter the state with an open mind and receive the therapist's suggestion. On a physical level, the only unusual feelings you may experience are a heaviness in your arms or a tingling in your hands and fingers.

After discussion of the techniques and procedures to be used in your case, the hypnotic sessions will begin. Generally, the hourly meetings will go something like this. You will enter a quiet room and be allowed to relax. Perhaps soft music will be played, or you will begin a previously taught method of relaxation. Sometimes the therapist will assist in the relaxation component of the therapy. Once you have achieved a calm state of mind and body, the therapist will begin a monologue that induces the hypnotic state. (This is the part of the session that most people think of when they envision hypnosis.) At this time, you will be told to continue to relax, or possibly to imagine a specific scene or experience a certain feeling. While the therapist speaks, you will become drowsy as your mind begins to let go of its focus on reality. Appraising your mental state and choosing the precise time, the therapist will begin a series of statements that are intended to correct negative thought patterns or to reinforce beneficial concepts and ideas. The session will end when the therapist requests you to respond to a specific statement or when you awake from a light sleep. For the most part, you will remember all that transpired.

As an example of an actual script, consider the following and try to get the feeling of a therapeutic session.

THERAPIST: I want you to sit back and relax. I want you to get as comfortable as possible and to close your eyes and relax. Relax and let your thoughts slip away. Take a slow deep breath and relax.

[*Pause*]

Now concentrate on your breathing. In long, slow, deep breaths, I want you to inhale. Inhale slowly, and let your lungs fill with air. Exhale. Exhale slowly, and allow your troubles to escape with your breath. Relax. Getting more and more comfortable now. Inhale. Exhale. Inhale. Exhale. Inhale and relax. Exhale completely and relax. More and more calm. More and more relaxed.

[*Pause*]

Now I want you to place your tensions and anxieties in a balloon. As I count from ten to one, let go of the balloon, and watch it sail away. Close your eyes and relax. Ten. Let go of the balloon. Watch it float away. Nine. Let go of the balloon, and watch it float away. Eight. Watch the balloon float away. Seven. Watch the balloon float higher and higher away. Six. It's getting smaller and farther away. Five. Watch the balloon float away. Four. The balloon is floating higher and farther away. Three. Watch the balloon float away. Two. Farther and farther away, smaller and smaller. One. Watch the balloon float out of sight.

[*Pause*]

Allow the image to fade, and concentrate on my words. Breathe yourself into a deeper state of relaxation. In and out. Slowly and deeply. Slowly and deeply. In and out.

[At this point or after a longer relaxation prelude, the hypnotherapist will create a therapeutic image or suggestion and will work with you for a while to ensure the incorporation of the thought into your mind and your memory. The suggestion might concern a particular problem you have expressed; it might relate to the treatment you are receiving, or perhaps to the direct destruction of your tumor. Sessions will vary, and suggestions will change according to your particular needs at the moment. Once the suggestions or images have been established, the therapist will bring you out of the hypnotic state.]

THERAPIST: Concentrate on what I have said. Allow those thoughts to reside deeply within your mind, constantly affecting the way you think and feel. Concentrate on what I have said, and allow those thoughts to work for you. Imagine yourself well. Imagine yourself healthy and well. Concentrate on those thoughts, and allow them to work for you. Carry these thoughts with you.

[Pause]

Now concentrate on your breathing. Slowly, deeply, breathe in and out. In and out. In and out. As I count from three to one, you will feel stronger and more alert. You will feel lighter and more awake. Three. Focus on my words and think about what I say. Focus on my words and think about what I say. Two. You are beginning to feel stronger and more awake. Stronger and more alert. One. Open your eyes slowly, and relax. Open your eyes slowly, and relax. Take a few slow deep breaths and relax.

[End of session]

Although the example just presented lasts only a few

minutes, it aptly conveys the feeling of a hypnosis session and also demonstrates the techniques used to bring on the hypnotic state and to generate the hypnotic suggestion. There are hundreds of variations on this theme; each therapist has a working script with which he or she feels comfortable. But the results of each script are the same—induction into a specific state of consciousness whereby certain suggestions can have a powerful effect on the way you think and feel.

On the surface, this may seem bland in comparison to other forms of therapy, but if you continue to apply the principles you learn, you will eventually notice a change in your thinking and in your attitudes. As you begin to understand and confront the psychological components of your illness, your innermost feelings will restructure themselves, the process that generated your tumor will begin to reverse. At this point, it is up to your immune system to take over. With the correct balance of mental and physical harmony, you will be well on your way to a complete recovery.

Remember that hypnosis in the treatment of cancer should be an elective part of a self-directed program used in conjunction with standard medical or surgical care. It should be initiated under the direction of a well-known and well-recognized psychologist or psychiatrist who has advanced training in the field and who has previously treated serious cases of mental and physical ailments, including cancer. Hypnosis should not be used as primary therapy, although in certain cases it would no doubt work well. Rather, it should become an intricate part of a well-designed adjunct program tailored to your specific needs. It is intended to give you a subconscious psychological edge in the fight against your illness.

Recommended Reading

Cheek, D., and L. Lecron. *Clinical Hypnotherapy*. New York: Grune and Straton, 1968.

Gibson, H. B. *Hypnosis: Its Nature and Therapeutic Uses.* New York: Taplinger, 1980.

Haley, J. *Uncommon Therapy.* New York: Norton, 1973.

Wolfberg, L. R. *Hypnosis: Is It for You?* New York: December, 1982.

HYPNOSIS FOUNDATIONS, SOCIETIES, GUILDS, AND ASSOCIATIONS

Academy of Scientific
Hypnotherapy
P.O. Box 12041
San Diego, CA 92112

American Guild of
Hypnotherapists
7117 Farnam Street
Omaha, NE 68132

American Society of
Clinical Hypnosis
2250 East Devon Avenue
Des Plaines, IL 60018

PSYCHOLOGY ORGANIZATIONS, SOCIETIES, AND ASSOCIATIONS

American Psychology
Association
1200 17th Street NW
Washington, DC 20036
202-955-7600

Association of Black
Psychologists
P.O. Box 55999
Washington, DC 20040
202-289-3663

International Council of
Psychologists
4805 Regent Street
Madison, WI 53705
608-238-5373

National Hispanic
Psychological
Association
P.O. Box 451 Health
2415 West 6th Street
Brookline, MA 02146
617-266-6336

National Psychological
Association
P.O. Box 2436
West Palm Beach, FL
33402
305-689-3787

Psychology Society
100 Beekman Street
New York, NY 10038
212-285-1872

Society for the
  Advancement of Social
  Psychology
Institute for Social
  Research
University of Michigan
Ann Arbor, MI 48109
313-763-2359

Society of Psychological
  Research
401 Parnassus Avenue
University of California
San Francisco, CA 94143
413-476-7622

For the names of psychologists in your area, consult:

American Psychology Association Directory. American
Psychology Association, 1985.

IV
COMBINING
THERAPIES

13
Metabolic Therapies and the Remission of Cancer

Cameron Stauth, in his dramatic book, *Alternative Cancer Therapies*, tells the amazing story of a thirty-four-year-old woman whose health had gradually deteriorated over several years. Starting with a protracted bout of bronchitis, which occasionally confined her to bed, she soon developed a constant wheeze and a chronic cough. At times she was too weak to do her housework or take care of her two children. In the years that followed, she saw the strength sapped from her once energetic body and in time fell into a deep depression that had replaced her normally cheerful personality. Ultimately, it became difficult to ascend a flight of stairs without resting for at least twenty minutes afterward.

Changes also occurred in her body during the five-year period. Due to a "lump" in her throat, swallowing became difficult, and the lump seemed to be ever increasing in size. Her nails, once hard and beautiful, gradually went brittle. The texture of her hair even changed. Obviously something was amiss, so she set an appointment to see her doctor.

On the first visit, her physician was not impressed by what she told him. As far as he was concerned, absolutely nothing was wrong with her, and there certainly was no reason for further tests or examinations. All she had to do was lose a few pounds, and everything would go back to normal. For the time being, she should simply endure her problems, and they would soon resolve.

While the young homemaker accepted this recommendation, her husband was less receptive and insisted that she consult another doctor. The second doctor was more concerned about the vague but unusual series of complaints, so he ordered x-rays and other tests. When the ominous results finally returned, another round of examinations and x-rays were immediately requested. Apparently there was a serious problem.

This time the young couple were called into the hospital to personally receive the results. The surgeon who supervised the testing did not have good news to report, so he took the husband aside to explain the problem in private. As he reviewed the x-rays, he pointed out a large mass in the lungs. He placed his fist over the dense chest lesion and shook his head in despair. "I'm afraid this is not a surgical case," he admitted, "the tumor is just too big; it's bigger than my fist."

"Tumor!" exclaimed the husband. That was the last word he had wanted to hear. How could it be? How could a woman so young have such a terrible illness? How could he tell her? What would he say?

"The x-rays are inconclusive, and a biopsy must be performed," was the way he broke the news to his anxious wife. He didn't have the heart to tell her outright.

They would have to wait a few days for the biopsy and a few more days for the results, but even then they really didn't know what they were dealing with. It wasn't until a second opinion was rendered by the pathology department at Stony Brook University that the diagnosis was established. The tumor was a hystiocytic lymphoma, the worst of all possible scenarios, carrying a prognosis of eight to ten months if treated, four to five months if left alone. Either way, the life expectancy was extremely poor, as the illness was almost always fatal following a rapidly debilitating course. Still, some form of therapy was needed if the woman were to have any chance of cure at all.

Radiation therapy was begun at Sloan Kettering Memorial Hospital in New York City, even though the attending physicians did not want to accept the case. After all, it had already been pronounced untreatable. But the husband's persistence forced the issue, and the young woman was prescribed a full course of therapy. In the beginning, she received 300 rads of radiation regularly in the hope of reducing the size of the tumors in her lungs and throat. This was absolutely necessary for her to continue to breathe and eat but extremely uncomfortable as well. The final treatment, consisting of 3,000 rads of radiation, left her weak and nauseated for days. In addition, her throat had been burned raw by the high intensity of the final cobalt treatment. Was it all worthwhile? Would this pain and suffering really alter the course of the disease? Only time would tell.

During the period of initial treatment, the husband spent much of his time researching the illness that had stricken his wife. He gathered as much information about hystiocytic lymphomas as he could find at the New York Academy of Medicine, but nothing provided much hope. Generally, patients with the disease live only about a year, and far-advanced cases, like his wife's, have an even poorer prognosis: four to six months is the rule. If only he could do something or take her somewhere, she would have a better chance of survival, he thought.

At about this time, a friend suggested that the husband look into metabolic therapies, naturalistic approaches to the treatment of cancer. In the academy's library, he was referred to the works of Linus Pauling on vitamin C and Max Gerson on holistic cancer therapies, but further information was lacking. He obtained other books on the subject and began to appreciate the innate ability of the body's own natural defense system to destroy cancer cells if given the chance through detoxification and stimulation of the immune response. He began to reason that if the results obtained by traditional methods of treatment of hysticocytic lymphoma were so poor, then his wife had little to lose if she tried alternative therapies.

So the husband began to provide her with vitamin C regularly and supplemented her diet with wholesome natural foods. He gave her some of the books he had bought so that she could familiarize herself with other ideas and forms of treatment. She was initially skeptical, coming from a long line of family members who thought that doctors could do no wrong and that unconventional forms of therapy were all unacceptable. Although disappointed, the husband didn't argue or try to force his views on his wife. Instead, he continued to quietly research other possible avenues of therapy and prepare himself for the change of treatment he thought was inevitable.

While helping his wife home from the hospital one day, the husband was confronted by the radiologist in charge of the case. The radiologist explained that the tumor had shrunk but was really expected to resume rapid growth in the near future. Chemotherapy would then be necessary to temporarily arrest the malignant spread that would ultimately take the woman's life, but it would at least prolong her life a few more months. With this news, the husband knew something else had to be done quickly. He made arrangements to visit a holistic physician in Washington State and prepared his wife for the journey.

Arriving at the small holistic center, they both felt as

if they had made a mistake. The center was small and looked unimpressive. It lacked the sprawling dimensions of Sloan Kettering and was even smaller than their local hospital. How could this structure house the medical talent necessary to cure patients of cancer? Were they right in seeking out this unconventional and out-of-the-way clinic? But their first visit with William Kelley, the director of the Kelley Foundation in Winthrop, Washington, put them at ease, and they decided to listen to what Dr. Kelley had to offer. It was a wise decision.

Dr. Kelley assured the two that he could help, but that it would take a lot of work because of the advanced state of the disease. He told his new patient that it was her responsibility to make herself well. She would have to fight for her health as she had done so many times before whenever she was ill—only this time it would require a totally dedicated effort and complete conviction. It was Dr. Kelley's opinion that the proper diet, nutritional supplementation, psychological therapy, internal purification, and lifestyle change could modify the immune system enough to thwart the disease, to reverse the horrible trend that had caused and carried the cancer to such a critical state. As it was for all of his patients, her case was unique and would require a special program, one tailored to her needs. He would provide such a program, but she had to abide by it if she were to succeed in her quest against her illness.

From the onset of treatments, the young woman began to feel slightly better. The soreness in her throat greatly subsided, as did the nausea that had plagued her since the radiation therapy. She found that the coffee enemas, which she had originally viewed as repulsive, worked exceedingly well in treating the nausea, so she employed the procedure whenever she felt queasy. Immediate relief always followed. Food supplementation, which she had first considered an inconvenience and a bother, became a welcome addition to her diet because of the strength and vitality it afforded. Liver and bile flushes noticeably detoxified her body, and a change in diet altered her body chemistry just enough to improve her moods and emotions.

A return visit to the doctor who had originally diagnosed the illness only complicated the picture, however. He didn't believe that adjunct therapies had a place in modern medicine. He belittled the holistic approach to the treatment of illness and firmly thought that in cases of cancer it was a complete waste of time. He insisted that "his" patient be placed on a chemotherapeutic program immediately, or else he could not assume responsibility for what was going to happen to her. If she wanted to kill herself with some silly program of internal cleansing, that was her business, but he wanted nothing to do with it. Chemotherapy or else was his position, and with that he dropped the case.

Now completely on her own, the courageous patient continued to apply the principles of holistic therapy with the help of her husband. She changed her entire lifestyle to accommodate the recommendations of the program that Dr. Kelley had given her, and with frequent phone calls to a holistic doctor in Connecticut, she made any necessary corrections. She spent much of her time during the day just preparing the foods she had to eat, juicing the fresh fruits and vegetables that formed such an important part of the diet, fixing her meals with precision. She continued to take the coffee enemas and to perform the flushes and purges that were vitally important to the purification of her liver and gastrointestinal tract. She exercised lightly to improve her strength and endurance and consumed dozens of food supplements daily. She improved physically and emotionally every day.

For months she kept up this routine with obvious benefit and overwhelmingly positive results, but then something happened. Quickly and unexpectedly, her condition again began to turn around. She began to feel worse. Fever ensued. Depression set in. She was confined to bed.

Her long-distance consultant, the Connecticut holistic physician, assured her that this reaction was to be expected. It was only a sign that the treatments were working. Since she had so aggressively attacked her cancer, its rapid destruction and elimination brought with them excessive toxicity that had overwhelmed her system and taxed her ability to dissipate the dead and dying cancer cells. She was instructed to exercise extreme caution not to stimulate her immune system so radically, because such stimulation could cause her death.

At this point, the woman just did not know what to think. Was the doctor just placating her? Was the therapy just a waste of time, as her Long Island doctor had so vehemently insisted? It was beginning to look that way.

With each passing day, her constitution deteriorated. Although still mentally tough, she had numerous physical setbacks, the most severe of which was sleep apnea, a condition in which she would actually stop breathing in her sleep. Every night, she would take an abrupt deep breath, emit a lengthy sigh, and then simply stop breathing. Her husband, who would sit through the nights with her, would have to stimulate her breathing with a blow to her back in order to get her lungs working again. The condition was as life threatening as it could be.

In desperation, they again consulted the Long Island doctor. This time he was angry and hostile. His appraisal of the situation was extremely grave, arguing that the tumor had enlarged to the point that it had impinged on her windpipe and was about to completely close off the air to her lungs. If chemotherapy were not started immediately, she would be dead within a matter of days. But the couple was still uncertain. They wanted to see for themselves exactly what was going on before they submitted to any other form of therapy. Was it the tumor compressing on the trachea that was causing the symptoms, or was radiation fibrosis of the lungs producing the sleep apnea? This question had to be answered before anything else could be done. The answer would signal the young women's fate. An x-ray was needed.

But the Long Island doctor would not order the x-ray. He was convinced that the problem was not fibrosis of the lungs, but rather the cancerous tumor, and he insisted again on the chemotherapy. His adamancy was unacceptable to the woman, so she sought help elsewhere. She instinctively turned to the Connecticut doctor who had been so understanding throughout the illness. She knew that she could count on him to do what she and her husband wanted, so they drove up to Connecticut for a series of x-rays—the results of which were unbelievable.

As the couple waited to speak to the radiologist who had taken the chest films, they sat in high anticipation. The report was too slow in coming. Good news travels fast, so the x-rays must be ominous, they both thought. When the doctor finally did appear, he had a horrible look on his face. With reluctance and difficulty, he expressed his great concern for the future of this young woman. As far as he could determine, it was one of the worst cases he had ever seen. Over 90 percent of the left lung had been lost to fibrosis. It was a very bad case.

The husband, less worried about the fibrosis than the cancer, quickly interjected: "But how large is the tumor?"

The new radiologist, not completely familiar with the case, was suddenly perplexed. "What tumor?" he replied. "There's no sign of tumor anywhere in these x-rays." Unaware of the patient's concern about her resolved cancer, he only saw and commented on the fibrous scarring that is a part of the healing process. In time, this too would resolve.

From this case, along with the others presented in this book, you see that healing can come unexpectedly, when all hope seems gone and the probability of recuperation is reduced to a thin thread of luck. Under these circumstances, you think that only a miracle could deliver you from your dilemma and pull you from the depths of illness and the grip of death. Then something happens that changes your fate, and in a trick of the tale, you are saved. Like an O. Henry story with an unexpected ending, your life is turned around. Through your will and the natural ability of your body, your illness vanishes, and you are given a clean bill of health.

In the case just presented, the critically ill woman placed her hope and faith in the self-administered therapies she learned from her holistic physicians. It took great courage and complete dedication, but in the end, the results were overwhelmingly worth the effort. She achieved the remission she so desperately sought.

The metabolic therapies used in the case were not new; they were developed over a period of two centuries by a host of physicians. First on the list of notable proponents was William Lambe, a British doctor who, early in the nineteenth century, published articles on the value of nutritional treatments in cases of malignancy. Later in that century in London, two other physicians, Waldon Fell and John Pattison, began to treat cancer with herbs and chemicals. Perhaps the most inclusive approach to the problem was advanced by Bob Bell and Forbes Ross, who thought that dietary modifications with an emphasis on specific nutrients could substantially alter the biochemical composition of the body and subsequently change the course of the disease.

In the United States, similar attitudes were brewing. Nutritional interest began to heat up considerably with the work of two physicians, Charles Ozias and Lucian Bulkley. By 1960 many holistic physicians, including Virginia Livington, Harry Hoxsey, William Koch, and the now well-known Max Gerson, were all creating metabolic programs that form the basis of treatments that are still in use today; all advocating the enhancement of the body's own natural defense system. These doctors believed that multiple stimulation of the many elements of the immune system could enable it to weaken and destroy tumor cells. They then showed that the combined use of internal cleansing and powerful diets could increase the effectiveness of organ function and bolster overall health to effectively eliminate the problem.

Today, several metabolic programs are in use throughout the world. In Mexico, throughout the United States, and in Germany and Austria, they are being used to help patients fight their cancers by combining conventional and unconventional treatments.

KELLEY'S NONSPECIFIC METABOLIC THERAPY

William Kelley, whom we discussed earlier in the chapter, has established a program called nonspecific metabolic therapy, which consists of three basic principles: direct destruction of cancer cells, strong therapeutic nutrition, and vehement detoxification. Dr. Kelley, along with the other researchers in the field, believes that malignancies arise from a malfunctioning pancreas and insufficient release of pancreatic enzyme. Dr. Kelley's conviction is that pancreatic enzymes are essential to the prevention, natural destruction, and elimination of cancer. In conjunction with the immune system, the enzymes digest cancer cells as they arise. However, when insufficient in quantity, the enzymes are rendered ineffective, giving tumor cells a chance to grow and circumvent the regular processes of eradication. This condition can be reversed through diet, nutritional supplementation, and internal cleansing.

Dr. Kelley's diet and the other aspects of his program

are specifically tailored to the individual needs of his patients. Still, common threads run through each individual therapy. For example, raw fruits and vegetables form a major part of the nutritional plan of each participant at his foundation. Protein consumption is greatly reduced in order to preserve the enzymes needed to digest this food group. Enzyme supplementation is promoted. Megadoses of vitamins and minerals are advocated.

Even with the use of nutritionally superior foods and large quantities of vitamins and minerals, the overall dietary program must be tailored to match the metabolic character of the patient. The program considers the individual's personality, physiology, neurologic and physical makeup, health, and basic metabolic rate. A computer analysis of these traits fits each person into a specific category. Based on the final classification, an explicit diet is coordinated with the metabolic type, in order to avoid any nutritional waste.

Combined with the diet are physical purges that cleanse the liver, gallbladder, intestines, kidneys, and lungs. Metabolic therapists contend that the function of these organs is greatly compromised in the cancer patient, and that without thorough cleansing, the probability of survival is severely limited. The cleansing tasks are accomplished through liver and gallbladder flushes, colonic irrigations, controlled sweating, and stimulation of the kidneys and lungs. Once the waste materials and toxins are removed, these organs will perform their vital functions more precisely and enhance the body's ability to rid itself of cancer. It is also thought that the toxins, long stored in the organs of elimination, are in part responsible for the actual development of the malignancy and help to sustain the unhealthy internal environment that supports the cancerous process.

The actual techniques of Dr. Kelley and his associates can be obtained directly from the Kelley Foundation and Clinic or from a complete book about his therapies entitled *The New Approach to Cancer*. Described in detail are the principles behind the treatments and the methods of accomplishing the dietary change, detoxification, structural therapy, emotional adjustment, and lifestyle modification. Some of Dr. Kelley's explanations of the causes of cancer are purely speculative, but this does not negate the therapeutic value of the complete program. These procedures are excellent tools for altering the various tissues and fluids in the body, and they aid in the destruction and elimination of cancer.

LAETRILE: ERNST KREB'S APPLICATION OF THE JOHN BEARD THEORY

John Beard theorized that cancer is the outgrowth of trophoblast cells residing within the various organs of the body. Somehow, these rapidly growing cells of the early human embryo/placenta escape destruction by the pancreatic enzymes of the fetus and survive for decades in the internal organs. Then, with a functional decrease in the enzymes of the pancreas later in life, these hidden cells spring to life, developing into a tumor.

On the basis of this theory, Ernst Kreb developed a natural substance, laetrile, to replace the deficient pancreatic enzyme, chymotrypsin. By combining with another enzyme, beta glucuronidase, laetrile forms a compound called hydrocyanic acid, which contains the poison, cyanide. In very small quantities, the cyanide is tolerated by normal cells, which have the potential to metabolize it; but cancer cells, which lack the necessary enzyme, rhodanase, cannot dispense with the cyanide and subsequently succumb to it. In other words, laetrile kills cancer cells but does not affect normal cells. This, at least, is the view of Ernst Kreb.

While hundreds, perhaps thousands, of reports have been published on laetrile's effectiveness (or lack thereof), no conclusive study has proved its performance. The U.S. Food and Drug Administration has never accepted the claims of success made by the supporters and users of laetrile, but that has not stopped the hopeful patients who have sought out this substance in foreign countries and clandestine clinics in the United States. If you feel that it will help in your case, by all means use it as an adjunct treatment but certainly not as a primary treatment. Remember, primary therapy should be reserved for procedures and medications that have been absolutely proven effective through years of study and clinical practice.

THE COMBINED CANCER PROGRAMS OF HANS NIEPER AND JOSEPH ISSELS

The program of Hans Nieper, the discoverer of vitamin B_{13}, is a combination of several metabolic cures that act together to destroy cancer. Dietary changes are instituted, and a mineral balance is supported by supplementation of phosphorus, potassium, iron, zinc, magnesium, and copper. (Interestingly, copper has recently been shown to slow the growth rate of cancer cells.) Dietary calories come primarily from whole grains, and the consumption of sugar, animal protein, and shellfish is strictly limited. The patient receives low doses of chemotherapy and radiation to achieve a balance between traditional and metabolic therapies. Dr. Nieper's patients stay in rooming houses or at his hospital just outside of Hanover, West Germany.

In the nearby town of Rottach-Egern, Austria, Joseph Issels's Ringberg Clinic provides the setting for another combined program of cancer therapy. Dr. Issels's approach is to eradicate malignancy through a combination of well-established therapies and less conventional cures. Surgery, radiation, and chemotherapy are used at appropriate times in the treatment of his patients, along with fever therapy and ozone infusion. The immune system is stimulated with dietary modification emphasizing whole grains and fiber, plus vitamin and mineral supplements, notably vitamins C, A, B complex, and E. To further enhance the immune system, patients participate in a daily exercise program that includes jogging and light mountain climbing.

Ozone and oxygen infusion therapy, fairly uncommon in the treatment of cancer, are performed in the following manner. The blood of the patient is cross-matched with donor blood that is then heavily oxygenated. This new cross-matched blood is transfused into the patient with the intention of destroying the cancer. The effect is threefold. First, the donor blood will contain a high level of oxygen, which is deleterious to malignant cells. Second, the white blood cells in the donor's blood may directly attack the tumor. Third, the mild transfusion reaction that is caused with any exchange of blood my further stimulate the patient's own immune system into increased action. To accomplish this same purpose, Dr. Nieper sometimes uses vaccines derived from the tuberculosis bacterium in order to bolster the natural defense systems of his patients.

Also noteworthy at the Ringberg Clinic is the use of fever therapy. Although Dr. Issel has proposed this type of treatment for twenty-five years, it has just recently won acceptance in the United States. Its new label is hyperthermia.

The rationale behind hyperthemia is that cancer cells are more heat-sensitive than normal cells. In fact, they cannot tolerate heat in excess of 107 degrees Fahrenheit. Stimulated or simulated fever causes the body temperature to rise and creates an unacceptable habitat for the cancer. Currently in the United States, hyperthermic units consist of body encasements through which circulates water heated to 113 degrees. While carefully monitored to prevent the untoward effects of prolonged exposure to such temperatures, the patient is gradually brought to about 107.5 degrees and held there for about two hours. During this period, intravenous fluids are constantly provided to balance the two quarts of water lost through copious sweating. A computer keeps track of all vital signs to assure a successful and safe outcome. Although the results of hyperthermic treatments are still being evaluated, the procedure has at least been proved safe and offers some promise.

THE THERAPY OF MAX GERSON

The metabolic approach to the treatment of cancer that has come to be relatively standard among holistic physicians is, in large part, the Max Gerson approach. During his life, Dr. Gerson researched and promoted the use of dietary and lifestyle changes as important components of the complete treatment of cancer. His findings have since stirred many other doctors and researchers to investigate the benefits of metabolic treatments in the care of their patients.

Gerson's work focused on the positive effects on the body's health and natural defenses that are achieved through therapeutic diets and physical detoxification. His personal dietary program consists mainly of vegetables, raw salads, and fresh fruits in salt-free, fat-free, and low-protein meals. At the top of the menu is a juice prepared from fresh carrots, green leafy vegetables, and baby calves' liver. Eleven glasses are required each day. The diet is supplemented with thyroid extract, potassium iodide, digestive enzymes, iodine, liver extract, and vitamins B_3 and B_{12}. Detoxification of the body is achieved with the previously mentioned coffee enemas. Later, this chapter describes how to prepare them.

During his lifetime, Gerson amassed volumes of research data and case histories indicating the effectiveness of the therapies he used. Acclaimed by some of the biggest names in medicine and panned by others, his work was constantly wrapped in controversy. Still, numerous intense efforts by the medical establishment failed to officially discredit his unconventional approach to the treatment of cancer, and untold numbers of patients have raved about his care.

The *Journal of Experimental Medicine and Surgery* (Volume 7, No. 4, 1949), describes one of his many successes. The patient's problem was diagnosed as a melanosarcoma of the left ankle, leg, and thigh, and she was operated on at Beekman Hospital in New York. Following a recurrence at the original sight with an extension to the lymph nodes, she underwent additional surgery at St. Luke's Hospital in New York, but in the end was given a hopeless prognosis because of the extent of the disease.

When the patient first saw Dr. Gerson she had a tumor described as "tomato-sized" in her left groin. The standard Gerson therapy of detoxification, nutrition, and supplementation was initiated on September 6, 1946. By June of the next year, no tumor could be found. In October 1948, the patient successfully delivered a healthy baby girl following uneventful pregnancy.

Max Gerson's accomplishments in the field of unconventional cancer therapy are world-renowned, and his techniques form the basis of most other metabolic or holistic approaches to the treatment of cancer. Since his methods are nonsurgical and employ only natural modes of healing, they can be used safely with all forms of traditional medicine and make excellent adjunct therapies.

THE PROGRAM AT AMERICAN INTERNATIONAL HOSPITAL

American International Hospital and its affiliated clinic are located in Illinois, about forty miles north of Chicago. Within its walls are practiced both traditional and unconventional therapies that have attained some of the highest success rates in the country. The hospital offers a combined program that assists in building up the patient's natural defense system through the use of vitamins, minerals, laetrile, and nutrition. Detoxification is routinely performed through the use of coffee enemas and the other methods previously discussed. Patients take pancreatic enzymes daily in high doses.

Other therapies used there include hyperthermia, aerobic exercise, prayer and spiritual development, short-term fasting, and the judicious use of surgery, chemotherapy, and radiation. As you can see, the program is well rounded to include major treatments from all fields of science and medicine, combined to suit the specific needs of the patient and to allow the doctor flexibility and creativity in choosing therapies. It is the future trend in the treatment of cancer and all other critical chronic illnesses.

METABOLIC OPTIONS

To review, take a look at this summary of the major components of some of the world's established metabolic programs.

Detoxification

Detoxification emphasizes the cleansing of the organs of elimination so that they can keep the body pure by effectively removing the toxins that cause and sustain cancer. There are many ways of accomplishing this, but here are some of the more common detoxification methods:

Colonic Cleansing (Coffee Enema)

Coffee enemas are highly stimulating to the liver, and help to remove built-up toxins and retained bile. The caffeine acts as a stimulant, and the procedure is also effective in reducing nausea.

1. Upon awakening in the morning, make a pot of regular, caffeinated coffee using a glass or Corning coffee pot or a drip system for purity. Use 1 to 4 table-

spoons of ground coffee per quart of distilled water.
2. Allow the coffee to cool to body temperature, and use it like any other enema, retaining the fluid for a total of fifteen minutes—five minutes while lying on the left side, five minutes while lying on the back, and five minutes while lying on the right side.
3. After the fifteen minutes, expel the fluid while rubbing the abdomen for complete elimination.

Liver and Gallbladder Cleansing

This procedure flushes biliary waste, including liver toxins and gallstonelike material, from the liver and gallbladder.

1. To soften gallbladder contents, drink plenty of fresh or organic apple juice and supplement with a phosphorus solution for five days. Individuals with problems tolerating fruit juice or sugar can simply take 90 drops of phosphorus solution each of the five days.
2. On the sixth day, two hours after lunch, consume 2 tablespoons of Epsom salts in a few ounces of mineral water.
3. Two hours thereafter, take a coffee enema with ¼ cup Epsom salts dissolved in it.
4. One hour thereafter, consume 1 tablespoon of Epsom salts in a few ounces of mineral water.
5. Two hours thereafter, consume a bowl of fresh fruit topped with heavy whipping cream.
6. Beginning two hours before bedtime, take 2 tablespoons of unrefined olive oil and 2 tablespoons of lemon juice every 15 minutes for 2 hours. (Nausea and vomiting sometimes occur.)
7. Go to bed and lie on your right side for at least 20 minutes with the right knee drawn to your chest before going to sleep.
8. Upon arising the next morning, take another coffee enema.

These wastes will subsequently appear in the stool as flecks of light to dark green material and green gelatinous matter.

Kidney Cleansing

1. The kidneys are easily flushed each day through the consumption of large quantities of water, herbal teas, and fruit and vegetable juices.
2. Watermelon juice also makes an excellent diuretic. Remove the fruit from the rind, juice it, and drink it.
3. In addition, twice weekly drink in the morning, the juice of 1 whole lemon in a glass of warm mineral water, followed by ten 8-ounce glasses of mineral water taken throughout the day. Constantly flushing the kidneys with pure water greatly reduces the concentration of the toxins generated by the tumor, the destruction of the tumor cells, and the therapies themselves. It also minimizes the harmful effects of these substances on the kidney tissue.

Purging

This procedure is excellent to cleanse the bowel and debride much of its contents. It is also an excellent way to increase your energy level and boost the effectiveness of the enzymes in your blood.

1. Upon arising in the morning, take a normal coffee enema.
2. One-half hour after elimination, take 1 tablespoon of Epsom salts dissolved in a few ounces of mineral water. Repeat two more times within the next hour.
3. Two hours thereafter, take a citric punch made from the juices of 6 lemons, 12 oranges, and 6 grapefruit mixed in 1 gallon of mineral water, one glass or more each hour throughout the day.
4. Repeat this procedure the next day and at least once every two months during your treatment.

These are just a few of the common procedures that metabolic doctors and holistic physicians use to cleanse and purify the physical systems of the body. These procedures should be conducted with the knowledge and recommendation of the doctor treating you. Their inclusion here is simply to familiarize you with some of the cleansing techniques so that you can better determine whether they are appropriate for you.

Nutrition

Extensive study of the relationship between cancer and food has shown that certain foods increase the incidence of malignancy, while others decrease the likelihood of ever developing the dreaded disease. An anticancer diet rich in grains, raw vegetables, and fruits breaks the cycle of poor nutrition and inadequate immune power. The patient in a metabolic program receives the nutritional means of support necessary to overcome his or her illness.

Supplementation

Elevated levels of vitamins and minerals have been shown to have a negative effect on cancer cells and a positive effect on longevity. Selective amounts of all vitamins and minerals are used in metabolic programs.

Enzyme Therapy

In theories developed over the past fifty years from studies on enzymatic destruction of tumors, it has been postulated that increasing the dietary intake of proteolytic enzymes causes increased enzymatic action to occur at the site of the tumor. This action greatly aids the components of the immune system, the white cells and the antibodies, in their never-ending struggle to overcome malignant forces in the body.

Laetrile

Use of laetrile is based on the fact that cancer cells are more sensitive to poisons than normal natural cells and do not possess the enzymes needed to metabolize the cyanide that is formed with the ingestion of laetrile.

Immunotherapy

A form of therapy alluded to in the case studies presented in Chapter 1, immunotherapy involves the administration of BCG, the bacterium used to form a vaccine against tuberculosis, in order to provoke an immune reaction against a tumor. It acts something like an anticancer vaccine and stimulates the forces of the immune system to be more aggressive in seeking out and destroying cancer cells.

The discovery that BCG injections have an anticancer potential was independently made by two well-known researchers, Bernard Halpern, who was working at the College of France, and Lloyd Old, who later became director of Sloan-Kettering Institute in New York. Further research was conducted around the world, and the use of BCG immunotherapy became standard practice in several medical centers. According to Lucien Israel, whose fascinating book *Conquering Cancer* makes excellent reading on the subject, the BCG stimulates macrophages to kill cancer cells. It apparently works best when combined with chemotherapy but has to its solo credit numerous cases of complete remission and innumerable cases of temporary or prolonged remission. It is used by traditional doctors as well as holistic physicians.

Traditional Therapies

Although some metabolic programs frown on the use of surgery, radiation, and chemotherapy, many modern facilities recognize the value of providing the full gamut of conventional and unconventional treatments.

The ultimate choice of adjunct treatment should be made by the patient, according to what he or she believes will be effective in his or her case. But adjunct therapies should be used only as they were intended, as *additions* to regular medical practices. With that in mind, the use of macrobiotics with supplementation is essential to the curative process, internal cleaning is also highly important, and all of the metabolic approaches have great merit. They offer a lifesaving power that should be combined with traditional treatments for a winning program, a total remission of cancer.

Recommended Reading

Bradford, R. W., with M. Culbert. *Now That You Have Cancer*. Los Altos, CA: Choice Publications, 1977.

Bricklin, M. *Natural Healing*. Emmaus, PA: Rodale Press, 1976.

Brody, J. with A. Holleb. *You Can Fight Cancer and Win* . New York: McGraw-Hill, 1977.

Culbert, M. *Freedom from Cancer*. New York: Pocket Books, 1976.

Deverell, D. *How I Healed My Cancer Holistically*.Manhattan Beach, CA: *Mother Earth News*. 1978.

Gerson, M. *A Cancer Therapy*. Del Mar, CA: Totality Books, 1958.

Glasser, R. *The Body Is Hero*. New York: Random House, 1976.

Haught, S. J. *Has Dr. Max Gerson a True Cancer Cure?* North Hollywood, CA: London Press, 1962.

Holzer, H. *Beyond Medicine*. New York: Ballantine, 1973.

Israel, L. *Conquering Cancer*. New York: Random House, 1980.

Kelley, W. *One Answer to Cancer*. Beverly Hills, CA: International Association of Cancer Victims and Friends, 1974.

Livingston, V. *Cancer: A New Breakthrough.* San Diego, CA: Production House Publishers, 1972.

Rapaport, S. A. *Strike Back at Cancer: What to Do and Where to Go for the Best Medical Care.* Englewood Cliffs, NJ: Prentice-Hall, 1978.

Stauth, C. *Alternative Cancer Therapies.* Brookline Village, MA: New Age, 1978.

HOLISTIC CENTERS GIVING REFERRALS

American Academy of
  Homeopathic Medicine
P.O. Box 75
Old Westbury, NY 07090

American Holistic Medical
  Association
Rural Route 2, Welsh
  Coulee
La Crosse, WI 54601

American Institute of
  Homeopathy
1500 Massachusetts
  Avenue, NW
Washington, DC 20005

Association for Holistic
  Health
P.O. Box 9532
San Diego, CA 92109

Canadian Holistic Healing
  Association
308 East 23 Avenue
Vancouver, BC Canada
  V5V 1X5

Coalition of Holistic Health
  Organizations
1424 16th Street, NW #105
Washington, DC 20036

Directory of Holistic
  Physicians
American Holistic Medical
  Association
6932 Little River Turnpike
Annandale, VA 22003

Hippocrates Health
  Institute
25 Exeter Street
Boston, MA 02116

Holistic Health
  Practitioners Association
396 Euclid Avenue
Oakland, CA 94610

Holistic Health Referrals
1 Brattle Circle
Cambridge, MA 02138

Holistic Health Review
72 Fifth Avenue
New York, NY 10011

Holistic Organizing
  Committee
P.O. Box 688
Berkeley, CA 94701

International Association
of Holistic Health
3419 Thom Boulevard
Las Vegas, NV 89130

International Foundation
for Homeopathy
2366 Eastlake Avenue East
Suite 301
Seattle, WA 98102

Life Force Cancer Project
2210 Wilshire Boulevard
Box 281
Santa Monica, CA 90403

Michigan Holistic Health
Association
P.O. Box 20082
Ferndale, MI 48220

National Council for
Alternative Health Care
P.O. Box 1132
San Jose, CA 95108

National Council on
Holistic Therapeutics
and Medicine
271 Fifth Avenue
New York, NY 10016

National Holistic
Federation
P.O. Box 688
Monrovia, CA 91016

Statewide Health Coalition
P.O. Box 1132
Jefferson City, MO 65102

Tri Self Clinic
510-14 Cornwall Avenue
Cheshere, CT 06410

Turtle Island Holistic
Health
569-71 Selby Avenue
St. Paul, MN 55102

Wholistic Health and
Nutrition Institute
150 Shereline Highway
#31
Mill Valley, CA 94941

IMMUNOLOGY CLINICS, CENTERS, PHYSICIANS

Nationwide: For a list of physicians and immunotherapists, contact:

Immunology Research
Foundation
70 West Hubbard Street
Chicago, IL 60610

Local

Yolanda Fraire, M.D.
P.O. Box 484
Coronado, CA 92118
619-488-4706
706-685-4665

Immunology Research
  Center
Lawrence Burton, Ph.D.
P.O. Box F 2689
Freeport, Grand Bahamas
809-352-7455/6

Virginia Livingston, M.D.
3232 Duke Street
San Diego, CA 92110
619-224-3515

Steenblock Medical Clinic
22821 Lake Forest Drive
Suite 114
El Toro, CA 92630
714-770-9616

LAETRILE THERAPY

Vera Allison, N.M.D.
4600 Kietzke Lane
Building B, Suite 112
Reno, NV 89502
702-826-8207

Ernesto Contreras, M.D.
Centro Medico del Mar
Paseo de Tijuana 1-A
Playas de Tijuana, Mexico
706-680-1203/4 or 1222
U.S. Contact:
P.O. Box 1561
Chula Vista, CA 92012
619-428-6438 (9-3, M-F)

Jan de Vries, Ph.N.D.
Auchenkyle Southwoods
Monkton, Ayrshire,
  Scotland
Troon 311414 (0292)

Harold Manner, Ph.D.,
  Director
Manner Clinic
Apartado 3437
Tijuana, B.C., Mexico
706-680-4422

U.S. Contact:
P.O. Box 4290
San Ysidro, CA 92073
706-680-4222 (reservations)
501-675-4962
305-454-8969

Hans Moolenburgh, M.D.
Oranjeplein II
Haarlem, Holland
023-316818

Manuel Navarro, M.D.
3553 Shining Morningside
  Terrace
Santa Mesa, Manila 2806
Philippines
2070-21 Local 391-47-21-
  51-55

Hans Nieper, M.D.
21 Sedanstrasse
3000 Hanover, West
  Germany
011-49-511-348-0808
(2-4 P.M., office)
011-49-5111-733-031
(9-11 A.M., hospital)

For more information, call the Hans Nieper Foundation: 714-2420-3775

Rosarita Beach Clinic (Tijuana, Mexico)
P.O. Box 5982
Chula Vista, CA 92012
706-689-4085 (Mexico)
619-426-2002

Salvadore Rubio, M.D.
(Tijuana, Mexico)
836 Orange Avenue, Suite 352
Coronado, CA 92118
619-575-6849

METABOLIC CLINICS, CENTERS, AND PHYSICIANS

Paul Beals, M.D.
9101 Cherry Lane, Suite 205
Laurel, MD 20708
301-490-9911

Brian Briggs, M.D.
718 6th Street, SW
Minot, ND 58701
701-838-6011

W. Douglas Brodie, M.D.
3670 Grand
Reno, NV 89509
702-825-2282

Dan Dotson, M.D.
921 4th Street
Graham, TX 76046
817-549-3663

Ray Evers, M.D.
Evers Health Center
P.O. Box 587
Cottonwood, AL 36320
205-691-2161
800-621-8924

William Faber, D.O.
6529 West Fond du Lac
Milwaukee, WI 53218
414-464-7680

Gerson Therapy
Gerson Institute
P.O. Box 430
Bonita, CA 92002

Bob Gibson, M.D.
215 North 3rd Street
Ponca City, OK 74601

Hoxley Therapy
Bio-Med Center
P.O. Box 727
Tijuana, B.C. Mexico

P. Jayalakshmi, M.D.
6366 Sherwood Road
Philadelphia, PA 19151
215-473-4226

Seiichi Kawachi, M.D.
7-3-8 Ginza Chuo-ku
Tokyo, 104 Japan
03-572-5455

Donald Mantell, M.D.
Preventive Medicine and Nutrition
6505 Mars Road
Evans City, PA 16033
412-776-5610

Harold Markus, M.D.
161 Avenue of the
 Americas
14th Floor
New York, NY 10013
212-675-2550

Irving Miller, N.D.
2613 North Stevens
Tacoma, WA 98407

W.W. Mittelstadt, D.O.
4001 North Ocean Drive
 #305
Ft. Lauderdale, FL 33308
305-491-4656

Preventive Medical
 Services
P.O. Box 82
Strathfield 2135
Sydney, Australia
02-764-4144

Owen Robins, M.D.
6565 De Moss, Suite 202
Houston, TX 77074
713-981-7500

Rodrigo Rodriguez, M.D.
American Biologics
 Hospital Mexico
(Tijuana, Mexico)
1180 Walnut Avenue
Chula Vista, CA 92011
619-429-8200

Ranulfo Sanchez, M.D.
American International
 Clinic
1911 27th Street
Zion, IL 60099
312-872-8722
800-367-4357

Michael Schachter, M.D.
Mountainview Medical
 Associates
Mountainview Avenue
Nyack, NY 10960
914-358-6800

John Sessions, D.O.
1609 South Margaret
 Street
Kirbyville, TX 75956
409-423-2166

Jack Slingluff, D.O.
5850 Fulton Road NW
Canton, OH 44718
216-494-8641

Nita A. Wolf, Director
Metabolics
P.O. Box 416
Wheatridge, CO 80033
303-233-1811/237-9006

14
Crossing the
Finish Line

Regardless of the type of cancer you may have or the seriousness of your condition, the decision to participate in your own treatment is probably the wisest decision you have ever made. It shows that you have a strong desire to affect the course of your illness, that you refuse to let your problems get the best of you, and that you are willing to fight to stay alive. This is the winning attitude required to beat cancer. It is the first commitment you needed. Congratulations; you're on your way.

Next is the selection of the therapy or therapies that will be most helpful in your cure. As you read through the information in this book about cancer and its creation, you no doubt could identify with many of the thoughts and concepts. You could probably see relationships between your experiences and the personal causes of cancer. While you may have just reflected momentarily on the topic during your reading, you must now precisely appraise what may have contributed to your illness, what created the negative environment that allowed your cancer to grow, and what habits or attitudes turned on your BAD SYSTEM. Think back for a moment. Maybe it was a diet high in calories and fat. It may have been a lack of exercise. Or maybe it was a poor mental attitude and prolonged states of depression or frustration. Perhaps too much stress was a factor. Whatever causes you can pinpoint, permanently record them now and use them as a guide in the selection of your adjunct treatments.

Once you have determined what contributed to your illness, rationally select the therapies that you believe will be of benefit in reversing your condition. For example, if you believe that a poor diet was the outstanding cause in your case, you might want to consider dietary therapy as an adjunct; if unexpressed emotions were a major factor, then a psychologically directed cure like hypnosis might be appropriate. The choices are up to you. But remember, select those therapies that you truly believe will be beneficial and that you feel you can adequately perform and uphold. After all, a half-hearted effort will probably only produce a half-hearted result, and in the case of cancer, that's just not good enough.

GETTING STARTED

The faster you make your selections and implement them, the better off you will be. Even if your doctor "thinks" the surgery, chemicals, or radiation "got it all," don't let that statement lull you into complacency. Apply the therapies of your choice to help ensure a total recovery. Even if your prognosis is excellent with traditional treatments and your cancer was discovered and treated in an early stage, don't think that you are out of the woods. Although you have an excellent chance of survival, you can better the odds by reversing the conditions that caused your cancer in the first place. Apply the adjunct therapies enthusiastically because your fight will be most easily won. Don't be lazy; cross the finish line and win the race.

In creating the proper program for you, it's probably wise to consider more than one therapy. Combine two or more for optimal benefit. This will maximize your efforts and put several factors to work in your behalf. Combinations that make sense are diet, exercise, and visualization; metabolic therapies, supplementation, and hypnosis; or meditation, purification, and exercise. Create combinations that are meaningful to you. What's more, if you believe that you can apply all of the therapies simultaneously, you should strongly consider doing so. The more, the better.

Next recognize that you will need assistance in order to achieve your goal of a complete and lasting cure. You will have to find the most competent physicians and therapists to help you meet and beat the challenge. The same rules apply to adjunct therapists as to traditional physicians—you need the best you can find. You will also need the cooperation of all those who will be working with you. Each doctor must be aware of your desire to receive the best care possible and your need to help yourself through your crisis.

In this area, you may meet some resistance. For years, traditional physicians have turned up their noses at any form of adjunct therapy. Likewise, most medical doctors used to be blind to the effects of diet on disease and even failed to see correlations between high-fat diets and heart disease or low-fiber diets and cancer of the colon. So too, were they blind to the association between exercise and illness, again failing to appreciate the wonderful benefit of aerobic activity in the correlation of all kinds of physical ailments. Of course, times have changed in these areas, and doctors now acclaim the benefit of diet and exercise on a wide variety of diseases. Unfortunately, many are still in the Dark Ages when it comes to cancer and adjunct therapies. In fact, some even refuse to consider the topic, just as they did in the past with concepts and principles that are widely accepted today.

Be prepared for such closed-mindedness, and establish a way of circumventing it. For example, explain to your primary physician that you are going to apply some of the modern forms of adjunct therapy in an effort to help yourself and to help his or her efforts on your behalf. Surely, the doctor should know by now that vitamin C in large doses has greatly helped cancer patients tolerate radiation and chemotherapy by dispersing and eliminating the toxins generated with these treatments. The doctor should also be aware of the advances in visualization and hypnosis that have proved to be boons for the cancer patient. Explain to him or her that you want to incorporate some of these self-directed programs into the treatment plan so that you can participate in your own cure and better your odds of survival. Also tell your doctor that it is extremely important for you to do so and that you would like him or her to share as much information as possible with the adjunct therapies you select. Remember, a positive, noncombatant attitude will probably ensure a positive, noncombatant attitude in return, so be respectful and tactful to achieve your goal of total cooperation from all parties.

The reverse is also important. Let it be known to your adjunct therapist that you expect full cooperation among all of the people who are involved in your treatment and that you want to achieve a balance of therapies that will be most beneficial to you. Like traditional physicians who criticize any unconventional approach to cancer treatment, some adjunct therapists are very opinionated about the benefits and hazards of traditional medicine. Some may even recommend that you completely abandon such treatment modalities as chemotherapy, radiation, or even surgery. This would be a big mistake, so you must explain to all your health care professionals that you want to combine the best of all worlds and need their help to do so. If you encounter any health care professional who is unwilling to cooperate with others working with you, or who refuses to adhere to your desires and wishes, simply seek out other help immediately before your total treatment plan is jeopardized.

In selecting your adjunct therapist, remember that all doctors are not created equal. Some are wiser than others, and some have better qualifications. With the exception of exercise therapists, meditation instructors, and possibly macrobiotics teachers, most of the physicians with whom you will work will be M.D.s, D.O.s osteopaths, or Ph.D.s. They should be well recognized by their colleagues, and they should have a wide range of experience in their chosen field. Publications and research in their respective specialties is also impressive. Equally important is their desire to help and the care and concern they project to you.

During your first session with a therapist, ask questions that can determine his or her competence. The doctor should meet your polite requests for credentials with a desire to inform you of schools attended and degrees held. A discussion of his or her experience should reveal numerous cases similar to yours, plus several years of practice in the field. A review of the results of these cases should be conservatively expressed yet convincingly positive. Finally, you should have a complete conversation about the projected approach of therapy in your particular case. In the end, you should feel confident and enthusiastic that you are about to begin a program that will be exciting, challenging, and extremely beneficial—actually lifesaving in your case. This is the attitude you must start with in order to achieve the best results, and your therapists should help create and perpetuate this attitude.

In the field of exercise and meditation, the qualifications of your teachers will be slightly different. Generally you will be working with instructors who respectfully want to aid in your physical and mental advancement. Exercise instructors, of course, must be knowledgeable in their field. In addition, they must be motivational in getting you to work out daily. You will be alone when performing much of your exercise—be it running, jogging, walking, or swimming. You therefore need to adequately understand the principles of aerobics so that you can properly perform your activity on your own. It is up to your instructor or doctor to teach these principles to you or to recommend sources of this information. (See the recommended reading in Chapter 9, "Exercise and the Remission of Cancer.")

If you choose meditation as an adjunct therapy, you must receive proper instruction from a yogi or other instructor at a recognized meditation center or perhaps in a course given at your local public school or at a nearby university campus. Once again, the instructor's role is to provide the techniques you will use in your meditation. He or she should also expand your awareness of yourself and your inner feelings and increase your appreciation of your place in the cosmos. The instructor will be your guide to new worlds within your consciousness, and he or she should eventually open new avenues of thought and experience. It is your job to apply this knowledge in your daily meditation and to constantly work with your instructor to increase the intensity of the process.

Most of the meditation instructors and yogis you will encounter are committed to a lifelong program of meditation and teaching. They are usually part of a specific group or foundation that not only teaches meditation but also instructs in a loving philosophy of life and a nonsectarian, nonreligious spirituality. They are seldom accredited professionals in the field of medicine, but they should have years of experience teaching meditation and also many dedicated students who will be learning with you. It is their purpose not to cure you of your illness—that's your job—but rather to change the way you look at things and to create an inner peace and harmony conducive to spiritual growth and self-healing. If you go to an accredited meditation course or established foundation, the instruction you receive will be adequate to get you started. The rest will be up to you.

Also of great importance in creating and perpetuating a positive, winning attitude is the support from family members and close friends. More than anyone else, these people can encourage you to keep going, to keep fighting even if the struggle gets tough. They are with you each day and can see the times when you most need encouragement. Their love and concern for your welfare can make the difference between success and failure, so inform them of your need for their assistance, and don't feel ashamed to call on them during your moments of need. They will be there to help.

REALISTIC GOALS

The road to remission may be long or short; regardless, you must travel it in order to reach the destination you desire. The journey requires dedication and work on your part, so prepare yourself well. Understand from the start that you will experience gains and setbacks. You will have good days and bad. But overall, your efforts will be rewarded.

With the use of the adjunct therapies, you will undoubtedly improve the quality of your life during the course of your illness. You will be more energetic and more vital than patients who just sit around waiting for nature to take its course. You will absolutely affect the course nature will take in your case, and you will affect it to the degree that you engage yourself in your selected adjunct program.

With adjunct therapies like macrobiotics, aerobic exercise, and metabolic purification, you should feel an immediate change for the better. If you select these therapies, you will undergo the fastest improvement of all, but understand that it will be difficult to initiate and maintain these programs. You will find that the diet is strict, the exercise is strenuous, and the metabolic purges are unusual practices. After the first day, you will be inclined to give it all up and take fate as it comes. But if you continue through the second day, you will be amazed that you had the willpower to do it, and you will feel a little stronger and a little more in control of your health. After the third day, you will begin to feel better than you have felt in a long time, and you will begin to develop a strength of mind and body that tells you that you are going to make it. If you can maintain your program of therapy for one week, you will understand the power that is at your command, and you will probably be able to continue for as long as it takes to achieve your goals.

Meditation, hypnosis, visualization, and other forms of biofeedback therapies that you might choose are more subtle, and noticeable results will take a little longer. This is not to say that they are less important than diet, exercise, or purification. It just means that they work in less obvious ways and have a less dramatic effect on your physical feelings and perceptions. Actually, they can be more specific and direct in attacking the cancer, because they are used to steer the forces of the immune system.

WHAT TO EXPECT

You can expect a variety of results from the adjunct therapies you choose. First, you will develop strength of character and be less prone to the feelings of despair and depression, helplessness and hopelessness that plague many cancer patients. Certainly you will not be helpless; after all, you are doing all the right things to assist yourself through your crisis. This dedication to your adjunct program creates the hope and faith that will keep you going, and as you continue with your therapies, integrating them into your life, you will carry an attitude of self-confidence and optimism that brings happiness rather than remorse to your daily living. You will feel better mentally and emotionally, knowing that you are doing everything in your power to beat your illness.

You can expect to feel physically better within a few days to a few weeks after initiating an adjunct program that includes either macrobiotics or exercise as one of its components. Of course, you will have up and down days, especially if you are receiving radiation or chemotherapy; this is to be expected. But you will be able to tolerate the traditional therapies better, and you will "bounce back" quicker with fewer down days.

You will get more out of the traditional therapies if you apply an adjunct program simultaneously. For instance, you can use visualization to increase the potency of radiation by envisioning the destruction of cancer cells as they are bombarded. You can also take high doses of vitamin C to protect normal cells and to accelerate the healing process once the radiation therapy is complete.

You will better the statistics for longevity and a total cure if you engage in a dedicated adjunct program. While it is impossible to predict with any degree of accuracy the exact number of patients who will experience a total and lasting remission through the combined application of both traditional and adjunct therapies, it is certain that the numbers are markedly skewed in your favor and that you will statistically outsurvive patients who make no attempt to employ therapies outside the scope of the big three—surgery, radiation, and chemotherapy. In addition, the quality of your life will be much enhanced throughout your illness, and you will be able to perform at a level approximately equal to 95 percent of your full capacity in all aspects of your daily living. If you incorporate aerobic exercise into your adjunct program, you will probably be more physically active than you were before your illness and might even achieve levels of daily performance above your previous capacities.

Finally, you will have something to work for. You will have a supreme goal to achieve, and you will have a definite and established way of reaching that goal. Unlike many cancer patients, who literally have nothing to do each day but worry about their illness, you will have a variety of planned activities that make each day interesting and challenging. You will have a positive mental attitude, vigor and vitality, physical activity, and perhaps even an elevated spirituality or ethereal view of life.

With these elements working in your favor, you will have the greatest of all possibilities of achieving a complete and total remission. So enter the race with confidence, give it your all for the last fifty yards, cross the finish on your own, and walk away a winner.

SUPPORT GROUPS AND CENTERS NATIONWIDE

Living with Cancer
P.O. Box 3060
Long Island, NY 11103

Make Today Count
343 East 23 Street
Brooklyn, NY 11226

Reach for Recovery
American Cancer Society
19 West 56 Street
New York, NY 10019

Holistic Health Support
245 East 77 Street
New York, NY 10001

INFORMATION NATIONWIDE

American Cancer Society
777 Third Avenue
New York, NY 10017

Cancer Counseling Center
29 Guentin Road
Scarsdale, NY 10583
914-723-8534

Cancer Information
Office of Cancer
Mayo Cancer Center
Rochester, MN 55905

Candlelighters
123 C Street, SE
Washington DC 20003

Center for Attitudinal
   Healing
19 Main Street
Tiburon, CA 94920
415-435-5022

Center for Medical
   Consumers
237 Thompson Street
New York, NY 10012

East West Holistic Center
141 Fifth Avenue
New York, NY 10010

Foundation for Alternative
   Cancer Therapies
Box HH Old Chelsea
   Station
New York, NY 10011

International Association
   for Cancer Victims and
   Friends
7740 West Manchester
   Avenue #110
Playa del Rey, CA 90293
213-822-5032

Mother Earth News
P.O. Box 70
Hendersonville, NC 28739

National Cancer Institute
Building #13, Room 10A21
National Institutes of
   Health
Bethesda, MD 20014

Tel-Med
P.O. Box 22700
Cooley Drive
Calton, CA 92324
Tapes via phone; call
   information for local
   telephone numbers

Treating Cancer
Consumer Information
   Center
Department 662 F
Pueblo, CO 81009

15
Another Winner

Dave Deverell, author of *How I Cured Myself of Cancer Holistically*, learned about her illness in 1972, when it was discovered that she had cancer in her breast, liver, stomach, pancreas, and groin. The discovery immediately prompted her to investigate the physical cause of the illness, which led her in turn to a study of the psychological and emotional states that help generate malignancies. She also investigated the nutritional aspects that cause and cure cancer.

With her new knowledge came the understanding that a tumor is really the physical expression of deeper problems—problems caused by emotional conflicts, poor nutrition, lack of exercise, and the like. She also realized that the outlook for the course of her disease was very poor if it were treated only with surgery, radiation, and chemotherapy. Resolved to treat the causes, not just the effects, she decided not to submit herself to surgery, radiation, or chemotherapy but, instead, to embark on a course of therapy that embraced more holistic treatments, which were designed to modify the personal causes of her disease.

In her case, she had to correct a poor self-image and the constant need for approval from others. She also had to stop feeling sorry for herself, to abandon the despair that had become an intricate part of her psyche, and to forgive and forget the injustices of previous years. She believed that a core of helplessness and hopelessness was at the center of her personality. It was fed by subconscious negative feelings that had to be discovered and dissolved before she could deal with her cancer.

The more she researched the personal causes of cancer, the more she identified with them. As she stripped away years of self-protective mechanisms, she began to uncover the deep emotions that had been suppressed for years—emotions so strong that they would have destroyed her ability to cope with life if they hadn't been suppressed. Unfortunately, the price she had paid for her previous false security was the cancer that grew throughout her body. She had cancer instead of emotional turmoil, cancer instead of self-acceptance. What a trade-off.

She decided that an appropriate course of therapy in her case had to be psychological, so she started to reprogram her emotions. In three sessions of fifteen to twenty minutes each day, she repeatedly told herself that she was no longer a child, that she was a mature adult capable of taking care of herself and able to do anything she set her mind to. She also practiced visualization in the form of a white light that radiated throughout her body, going to all the cancer sites and destroying all of the malignant cells.

To combine metabolic and psychological therapies, she subscribed to the program described in a book by William Kelley. Called *One Answer to Cancer*, it instructed her in the use of detoxification to cleanse the body of the harmful toxins that produce cancer and the nutrition that helps patients rid themselves of their malignant disease. Applying the information to her own life, she began to eliminate the poisons in her system with deep breathing, coffee enemas, saunas, fasting, and exercise. She became a vegetarian and removed even poultry, fish, and most dairy products from her diet. All processed foods were eliminated, along with cigarettes, alcohol, white flour, sugar, and caffeine. She started nutritional supplementation with hydrochloric acid tablets, minerals, vitamin E, vitamin C, vitamin A, vitamin D, high-potency B complex vitamins, pancreatic enzyme, desiccated liver, and predigested protein.

Her routine went something like this: About thirty minutes before breakfast, she would consume one teaspoon of chia seed that had been soaked overnight in fresh grape juice. For breakfast she ate raw cereal composed of a variety of grains, beans, and seeds combined with raisins or dates for sweetness. Apricot kernels and almonds were taken with a teaspoon of acidophilus bacteria, the lactobacillus used to make yogurt. Following her breakfast, she would stimulate and purge her system with a coffee enema.

A midmorning break for energy included the juice from two oranges, one grapefruit, and one lemon combined in an equal amount of water.

Lunch consisted of a fresh fruit salad, yogurt, ground sesame seeds, and more almonds, followed later in the afternoon by fresh carrot and celery juice.

Finally, for dinner she would have a green salad with sunflower, sesame, and pumpkin seeds. Whole-grain bread and sesame seed spread would complete the meal.

For thirty days she kept a rigid schedule of diet and detoxification, but thereafter she cut down the coffee enemas to twice weekly. After nine months, vitamin supplementation was also reduced to only vitamins C, E, B, A, and D. She continued her excellent dietary habits, and aerobic exercise remained an important part of her daily routine.

Slowly she began to feel better physically and mentally as she took control of her life. By maintaining her diet, she proved to herself that she had the power to direct life events. Through exercise she brought herself to a superior state of physical health. In time, she began to think and feel better than ever. She could sense that the effects were not only cumulative, but also self-stimulating, building on each other with each passing day. The core of helplessness and hopelessness soon dissipated, and her symptoms began to disappear.

After several more months, she went to see her nutritional doctor, who examined her and ran some tests to determine her overall state of health and the disposition of her cancer. To her dismay, she learned that she was still in a toxic state, as reflected by the results of her blood tests. But to her delight, she was in remission. There was no sign of cancer.

Later she admitted that she really wasn't surprised. She believed in the theories of Max Gerson, who maintained that recovery from cancer is possible if 50 percent of the function of the vital organs is intact. To her, it was a relatively simple matter to reverse the malignant process, but she conceded that it does take time, discipline, and plenty of hard work.

Today, she continues to take care of her mind and body by eating only the purest foods and running or swimming regularly. She controls herself and her mind through positive thinking and visualization. In addition, she has learned the most important lesson of all: that she is responsible for her own health and life, that she can direct life events through her dedicated efforts, and that life itself is given to those who aggressively go after it, to those courageous few who enter the race and give it their all for the last fifty yards. She was one of them, one of the winners.

Bibliography

CHAPTER 1, THE SPONTANEOUS REMISSION OF CANCER

Bluming, A. Z., and J. L. Zeigler. Regression of Burkitt's Lymphoma in Association with Measles Infection. *The Lancet* (1971): 105-106.

Boyd, W. *The Spontaneous Regression of Cancer*. Springfield, IL: Charles C. Thomas, 1966.

Everson, T. C., and W. H. Cole. *Spontaneous Regression of Cancer*. Philadelphia, PA: W. B. Saunders Co., 1966.

Franklin, C. I. V. Spontaneous Regression of Metastases from Testicular Tumours: A Report of Six Cases from One Center. *Clinical Radiology* 28 (1977): 499-502.

McSweeney, W. J., et al. Spontaneous Regression of a Putative Childhood Hepatoma. *American Journal of Diseases of Childhood* 125 (1973): 596-98.

Rosenberg, S. A., et al. Spontaneous Regression of Hepatic Metastases from Gastric Carcinoma. *Cancer* 29 (1972): 472-74.

CHAPTER 2, THE PROCESS OF HEALING

Bradbury, W., ed. *Into the Unknown*. Pleasantville, NY: Readers Digest Association, 1981.

Carrel, A. *Man the Unknown*. New York: Harper and Row, 1935.

CHAPTER 3, CONVENTIONAL THERAPY

American Medical Directory. 28th ed. 4 vols. Chicago: American Medical Association, 1982.

Crile, G. Jr. *Surgery: Your Choices, Your Alternatives*. New York: Delacoute, 1978.

Directory of Medical Specialists. 21st ed. 2 vols. Chicago: Marquis, 1983.

Lemaitre, G. D. *How to Choose a Good Doctor*. Andover, MA: Andover Publishing Group, 1979.

Morra, M. and E. Potts. *Choices: Realistic Alternatives in Cancer Treatments*. New York: Avon, 1980.

Salsbury, K. H. and E. L. Johnson. *The Indispensable Cancer Handbook: A Comprehensive, Authoritative Guide to the Latest and Best in Diagnosis, Treatment, Care, and Supportive Services*. New York: Wideview, 1981.

CHAPTER 4, WHAT YOU NEED TO KNOW ABOUT CANCER

Burnet, F. N. Cancer: Somatic-Genetic Considerations. *Advances in Cancer Research* 28 (1978).

Fink, D. J. Cancer Overview. *Cancer Research* 39 (1979): 2,819–21.

Guyton, A. C. *Textbook of Medical Physiology*. 4th ed. Philadelphia: W. B. Saunders Co. 1971.

Hick, R. Pathological and Biological Aspects of Tumour Promotion. *Carcinogenesis* 4 (1983): 1209–14.

Slaga, T. A., A. Sival and R. K. Boutwell, ed. *Carcinogenesis—A Comprehensive Survey*. Vol. 2, *Mechanisms of Tumor Promotion and Cocarcinogenesis*. New York: Raven Press, 1978.

Sutton, A., et al. Valine-Resistant *Escherichia coli* K-12 Strains with Mutations in the ilvB Operon. *Journal of Bacteriology*, (1981): 148, no. 3, 998–1001.

CHAPTER 5, THE NATURAL DEFENSE SYSTEM

Bennett, B., L. J. Old, and E. A. Boyse. The Phagocytosis of Tumor Cells in Vitro. *Transplantation:* 2 2 (1964): 183–202.

Burke, D. C. The Status of Interferon. *Scientific American* 256 (1977): 42–50.

Chany, C., et al. Constitutioning and Functioning of the Cell Membrane-Bound Interferon Receptor System. *Symposium on Interferons and the Control of Cell-virus Interactions*, Rehovot, Israel, 1977.

Gobel, U., et al. Comparison of Human Fibroblast and Leukocyte Interferon in the Treatment of Severe Laryngeal Papillomatosis in Children. *European Journal of Pediatrics* 137 (1981): 175–76.

Gresser, I. Antitumor Effects of Interferon. In *Cancer: A Comprehensive Treatise* edited by F. Becker. Vol. 5. New York: Plenum, 1973.

—— On the Varied Biological Effects of Interferon. *Cell Immunology* 34 (1977): 406–415.

Herberman, R., et al. Natural Killer Cells: Characteristics and Regulation of Activity. *Immunological Review* 44 (1979): 43–67.

Isaacs, A. Interferon. *Scientific American* 204 (May 1961): 51–57.

Isaacs, A. and J. Lindermann. Virus Interference: I. The Interferon. *Proceedings of the Royal Society of Serology and Bacteriology* 147 (1957): 258.

Key, M. and J. S. Haskill. Immonohistologic Evidence for the Role of Antibody and Macrophages in the Regression of the Murine T1699 Mammary Adenocarcinoma. *International Journal of Cancer* 28 (1981): 225–36.

McDaniel, M. C. Human Macrophage Activation Factors. *Inflammation*, 4 (1980): 125–135.

Padovan, I., et al. Effect of Interferon in Therapy of Skin, and Head and Neck Tumors. *Journal of Cancer Research and Clinical Oncology* 100 (1981): 295–310.

Strander, H. Interferons: Anti-Neoplstic Drugs: *Blut* 35 (1977): 277–88.

Strander, H., K. E. Morgansen, and K. Cantell. Production of Human Lymphoblastoid Interferon. *Journal of Clinical Microbiology* 1 (1975): 116–117.

Santoli, D. and H. Kaprowski. Mechanisms of Activation of Human Natural Killer Cells Against Tumor and Virus-Infected Cells. *Immunology Review* 44 (1979): 125–63.

Tadashi, S., et al. Effects of Intralesional Interferon on Neuroblastoma: Changes in Histology and DNA Content Distribution of Tumor Masses. *Cancer* 48 (1981): 2143–46.

Wheelock, E. F., and W. A. Sibley. Circulating Virus, Interferon and Antibody After Vaccination with the 17-D Strain of Yellow-Fever Virus. *New England Journal of Medicine* 273 (1965): 194.

CHAPTER 6, THE LINK BETWEEN THE MIND AND THE BODY

Achterberg, J. *Imagery in Healing.* Boston: New Science Library, 1985.

Benson, H. *The Relaxation Response.* New York: Morrow 1975.

Cousins, N. *Anatomy of an Illness as Perceived by the Patient. Reflections on Healing and Regeneration.* New York: W. W Norton, 1979.

Glasser, R. *The Body Is Hero.* New York: Random House 1976.

Green, E. E., A. M. Green, and E. D. Walters. Voluntary Control of Internal States: Psychological and Physiological. *Journal of Transpersonal Psychology* 11 (1970): 1–26.

Holmes, T. H., and R. H. Rahe. The Social Readjustment Rating Scale. *Journal of Psychosomatic Research* 11 (1967) 213–18.

Kissen, D. M. *Aspects of Neoplastic Disease.* Philadelphia PA: Lippincott, 1963.

Klein, A. Does Endogenous Cortisol Play a Role in the Development of Cancer? *Medical Hypotheses* 81 (1982): 163–71.

Kohler, G., M. Kohler, A. Satillaro, et al. *Healing Miracles Through Macrobiotics*. New York: Prentice Hall, 1982.

Kowal, S. J. Emotions as a Cause of Cancer. *Psychoanalytic Review* 42 (1955): 217-27.

LeShan, L. L. Psychological States as Factors in the Development of Malignant Disease: A Critical Review. *Journal of the National Cancer Institute* 22 (1959): 1-18.

—— *You Can Fight for Your Life*. New York: M. Evans and Co., 1977.

LeShan, L. L., and R. E. Worthington. Personality as a Factor in the Pathogenesis of Neoplastic Disease: A Review of the Literature. *British Journal of Medical Psychology* 29 (1956): 49-56.

Norris, P.A. *The Role of Psychophysiologic Self-Regulation in the Treatment of Cancer: A Narrative Report*. Topeka, KS: The Menninger Foundation.

Pelletier, K. *Mind as Healer, Mind as Slayer*. New York: Dell, 1977.

Reyher, J. Spontaneous Visual Imagery: Implications for Psychoanalysis, Psychopathology and Psychotherapy. *Journal of Mental Imagery* 2 (1977): 252-75.

Samuels, M., and H. Bennett. *The Well Body Book*. New York: Random House-Bookworks, 1973.

Samuels, M., and N. Samuels. *Seeing with the Mind's Eye*. New York: Random House-Bookworks, 1975.

Sapse, A. T. Stress, Cortisol, Interferon and "Stress" Diseases. *Medical Hypotheses* 13 (1984): 31-44.

Schmale, A. H., and H. Iker. The Psychological Setting of Uterine Cervical Cancer. *Annals of the New York Academy of Science* 125 (1966): 807-13.

Selye, H. *The Stress of Life*. New York: McGraw-Hill, 1956.

Sheikh, A., ed. *Imagery: Current Theory, Research and Application*. New York: Wiley, 1978.

Simonton, O. C., S. Simonton, and J. Creighton. *Getting Well Again*. Los Angeles: Tarcher, 1978.

Solomon, G. F., and R. H. Moos. Emotions, Immunity and Disease. *Archives of General Psychiatry* 11 (1964): 655.

Stephenson, J. H., and W. J. Grace. Life Stress and Cancer of the Cervix. *Psychosomatic Medicine* 16 (1954): 287.

Walshe, W. H. *Nature and Treatment of Cancer*. London: Taylor & Wallan, 1846.

Weatherhead, L. D. *Psychology, Religion and Healing*. New York: Abingdon-Cokesbury Press, 1951.

CHAPTER 7, MACROBIOTICS AND THE REMISSION OF CANCER

Kohler, G. M. Kohler, A. Satillaro, et al *Healing Miracles through Macrobiotics*. New York: Prentice Hall, 1982.

Kushi, M. *Cancer Prevention Diet*. New York: St. Martin's Press, 1983.

Kushi, M. and A. Kushi. *The Book of Macrobiotics*. Tokyo, Japan: Japan Publications, 1977.

Satillaro, A. *Recalled by Life*. Boston, MA: Houghton-Mifflin, 1982.

Wood, E. M. and C. P. Larson. Hepatic Carcinoma in Rainbow Trout. *Archives of Pathology* 71 (1961): 471–79.

CHAPTER 8, NUTRITIONAL SUPPLEMENTATION AND THE REMISSION OF CANCER

Adams, R. and F. Murray. *Improving Your Health with Vitamin C*. New York: Larchmont Books, 1978.

Bartlett M. K., C. M. Jones, and A. E. Ryan. Vitamin C and Wound Healing, II. Ascorbic Acid Content and Tensile Strength of Healing Wounds in Human Beings. *New England Journal of Medicine* 226 (1942): 474–81.

Bourne, G. H. Vitamin C and Immunity. *British Journal of Nutrition* 2 (1949): 346–56.

——. The Effect of Vitamin C on the Healing of Wounds. *Proceedings of the Nutrition Society* 4 (1946): 204–211.

Boyd, M. S. Can Garlic Lick Cancer? *Health* Vol. 19 no. 8 (1987): 13.

Cameron, E. and A. Campbell. The Orthomolecular Treatment of Cancer, II. Clinical Trial of High-Dose Ascorbic Supplements in Advanced Human Cancer. *Chemical-Biological Interactions* 9 (1974): 285–315.

Cameron, E. and L. Pauling. *Cancer and Vitamin C*, Menlo Park, CA: Linus Pauling Institute for Science and Medicine, 1979.

———. Supplemental Ascorbate in the Supportive Treatment of Cancer: Prolongation of Survival Times in Terminal Human Cancer. *Proceedings of the National Academy of Sciences USA* 73 (1976): 3685–89.

Cheraskin, E. and W. M. Ringsdorf. *New Hope for Incurable Disease.* New York: Arco, 1971.

Cottingham, E. and C. A. Mills. Influence of Temperature and Vitamin Deficiency upon Phagocytic Functions. *Journal of Immunology* 47 (1943): 493–502.

Dallin, L. *Cancer Causes and Controls.* Port Washington, NY: Ashley Books Inc., 1983.

Goetzl, E. J., S. I. Wasserman, I. Gigli, and K. F. Austen. Enhancement of Random Migration and Chemotactic Response of Human Leukocytes by Ascorbic Acid. *Journal of Clinical Investigation* 53 (1974): 813–18.

Kaufman, W. Niacinamide. A Most Neglected Vitamin. *International Academy of Preventive Medicine* 8 (1983): 5–25.

———. The Use of Vitamin Therapy to Reverse Certain Concomitants of Aging. *Journal of the American Geriatrics Society* 3 (1955): 927–36.

Mayer, J. A. *Diet for Living.* New York: Pocket Books, 1977.

McCormic, W. J. Cancer, a Collagen Disease, Secondary to a Nutritional Deficiency. *Archives of Pediatrics* 76 (1959): 166–71.

Mindell, E. *Vitamin Bible.* New York: Rawson-Wade, 1979.

Passwater, R. A. *Cancer and Its Nutritional Therapies.* New Canaan, CT: Pivot Original Health Books, 1978.

———. *Supernutrition.* New York: Dial Press, 1975.

————. *Supernutrition: Megavitamin Revolution*. New York: Pocket Books, 1976.

Pfeiffer, C. C. *Zinc and Other Micro-Nutrients*. New Canaan, CT: Keats Publishing, 1978.

Pritikin, N. *The Pritikin Promise: 28 Days to a Longer, Healthier Life*. New York: Simon and Schuster, 1983.

Rivici, E. A New Concept of the Pathophysiology of Cancer. *Psychosomatic Medicine* 19 (1957): 409–418.

Schwerdt, P. R., et al. Effects of Ascorbic Acid on Rhinovirus Replication in WI-38. *Proceedings of the Society for Experimental Biology and Medicine* 148 (1975): 1237–43.

Shute, W. E. *The Complete Updated Vitamin E Book*, New Canaan, CT: Keats Publishing, 1975.

Sporn, M. Role of Retinoids in Differentiation and Carcinogenesis. *Cancer Resident* 43 (1983): 3034–40.

Stone, I. *The Healing Factor: Vitamin C Against Disease*. New York: Grosset & Dunlap, 1972.

Williams, R. J. *Nutrition Against Disease*, New York: Pitman, 1971.

CHAPTER 9, EXERCISE AND THE REMISSION OF CANCER

Barry, A. J. Physical Activity and Psychic Stress/Strain. *Canadian Medical Association Journal* 96 (March 25, 1967): 848–51.

Cooper, K. *Aerobics* New York: Bantam, 1968.

Ewing, *Causation, Diagnosis and Treatment of Cancer*. Baltimore, MD: Williams & Wilkins Co., 1931.

Glassford, R. G., G. H. Y. Baycroft, A. W. Sedgwick, and R. B. J. MacNab. Comparison of Maximal Oxygen Uptake Values Determined by Predicted and Actual Methods. *Journal of Applied Physiology* 20 (May 1965): 509–13.

Grimby, G., N. J. Nilsson, and B. Saltin. Cardiac Output During Submaximal and Maximal Exercise in Active Middle-Aged Athletes. *Journal of Applied Physiology* 21 (July 1966): 513–26.

Ioffman, S. A. and K. E. Hoffman, Paschikis, et al. The Influence of Exercise on the Growth of Transplanted Rat Tumors. *Cancer Patient* 22 (1962): 597–99.

Knehr, C. A., D. B. Dill, and W. Neufeld. Training and Its Effects on Man at Rest and at Work. *American Journal of Physiology* (March 1941): 209.

Kraus, H., and W. Raab. *Hypokinetic Disease-Diseases Produced by Lack of Exercise* Springfield, IL: Charles C. Thomas, 1961.

Newton, J. L. The Assessment of Maximal Oxygen Intake. *Journal of Sports Medicine* 3 (June-September 1963): 165–69.

Roskamm, H. Optimum Patterns of Exercise for Healthy Adults. *Canadian Medical Association Journal* 96 (March 25, 1967): 890–98.

CHAPTER 10, MEDITATION AND THE REMISSION OF CANCER

Alexander, F. *Psychosomatic Medicine.* New York: W. W. Norton, 1950.

Allison, J. Respiration Changes During Transcendental Meditation. *The Lancet,* 1 (1970): 833–34.

Bagchi, B. K., and M. A. Wanger. *Electroencephalography, Clinical Neurophysiology and Epilepsy,* vol 3. London: Perganon, 1959.

Blumberg, E. T., R. M. West, and F. W. Ellis. A Possible Relationship Between Psychological Factors and Human Cancer. *Psychosomatic Medicine* 16 (1954): 277–90.

Brosse, T. A. Psychophysiological Study. *Main Currents in Modern Thought* 4 (1946): 77–84.

Brown B. *New Mind, New Body.* New York: Harper and Row, 1975.

Domash, L., J. Farrow, and D. Orme-Johnson. *Scientific Research on Transcendental Meditation.* Los Angeles: Maharishi International University, 1976.

Dunbar, F. *Emotions and Bodily Changes.* New York: Columbia University Press, 1954.

Eliasberg, W. G. Psychotherapy in Cancer Patients. *Journal of the American Medical Association* 147 (1951): 525-26.

Evans, E. A. *A Psychological Study of Cancer*. New York: Longman, 1928.

Fisher, S., and S .E. Cleveland. Relationship of Body Image to Site of Cancer. *Psychosomatic Medicine* 18 (1956): 304-309.

Goleman, D. Meditation and Consciousness: An Asian Approach to Mental Health. *American Journal of Psychotherapy*. 30, no. 1 (1976): 41-54.

Goleman, D. and G. E. Schwartz. Meditation as an Intervention in Stress Reactivity. *Journal of Consulting and Clinical Psychology*. 44 (1976): 456-66.

Greene, W. A., Jr. The Psychosocial Setting of the Development of Leukemia and Lymphoma. *In Psychophysiological Aspects of Cancer*. New York: New York Academy of Sciences, 1966.

Holmes, T. H., and M. Masuda. Life Change and Illness Susceptibility, Separation and Depression. *American Academy of Arts and Sciences* 5 (1973): 161-86.

Kasamatsu, A., and T. Hirai. Studies of EEGs of Expert Zen Meditators. *Folia Psychiatrica Neurologica Japanica* 28 (1966): 313-15.

Leizon, K. Spontaneous Disappearance of Bilateral Pulmonary Metastases: Report of Case of Adenocarcinoma of Kidney After Nephrectomy. *Journal of the American Medical Association* 169 (1959): 1737.

LeShan, L. E. Personality as a Factor in the Pathogenesis of Cancer: A Review of the Literature. *British Journal of Medicine and Psychology* 29 (1956): 49-56.

Meares, A. Stress, Meditation and the Regression of Cancer. *The Practitioner* 226 (1982): 1607-10.

Pelletier, K. R. *Mind as Healer, Mind as Slayer*. New York: Dell, 1977.

Pitts, F. N., Jr., and J. N. McClure, Jr. Lactate Metabolism in Anxiety Neurosis. *New England Journal of Medicine* 277 (1967): 1329-34.

Selye, H. *The Physiology and Pathology of Exposure to Stress.* Montreal: Acta, 1950.

Solomon, G. F. Emotions, Stress, the Central Nervous System, and Immunity. *Annals of the New York Academy of Science.*164 (1969): 335-43.

Wallace, R. K. Physiological Effects of Transcendental Meditation. *Science* 167 (1970): 175-54.

Wallace, R. K. and H. Benson. The Physiology of Meditation. *Scientific American* 22 (1972): 85-91.

CHAPTER 11, VISUALIZATION AND THE REMISSION OF CANCER

Achterberg, J. *Imagery in Healing.* Boston: New Science Library, 1985.

Benson, H. *The Relaxation Response.* New York: Morrow, 1975.

Holmes, T. H., and R. H. Rahe. The Social Readjustment Rating Scale. *Journal of Psychosomatic Research,* 11 (1967): 213-18.

LeShan, L. L. Psychological States as Factors in the Development of Malignant Disease: A Critical Review. *Journal of the National Cancer Institute* 22 (1959): 1-18.

———. *You Can Fight for Your Life.* New York: M. Evans and Company, 1977.

LeShan, L. L., and R. E. Worthington. Personality as a Factor in the Pathogenesis of Neoplastic Disease: A Review of the Literature. *British Journal of Medical Psychology* 29 (1956): 49-56.

Norris, P. A. *The Role of Psychophysiologic Self-Regulation in the Treatment of Cancer: A Narrative Report.* Topeka, KS: The Menninger Foundation.

Reyher, J. Spontaneous Visual Imagery: Implications for Psychoanalysis, Psychopathology and Psychotherapy. *Journal of Mental Imagery* 2 (1977): 252-75.

Samuels, M., and H. Bennett. *The Well Body Book.* New York: Random House-Bookworks, 1973.

Samuels, M., and N. Samuels. *Seeing with the Mind's Eye*. New York: Random House-Bookworks, 1975.

Selye, H. *The Stress of Life*. New York: McGraw-Hill, 1956.

Sheikh, A., ed. *Imagery: Current Theory, Research and Application*. New York: Wiley, 1978.

Simonton, O. C., S. Simonton, and J. Creighton. *Getting Well Again*. Los Angeles: Tarcher, 1978.

Trestman, R. L. *Imagery, Coping and Physiological Variables in Adult Cancer Patients*. The University of Tennessee, Knoxville, 1981.

Weatherhead, L. D. *Psychology, Religion and Healing*. New York: Abingdon-Cokesbury Press, 1951.

CHAPTER 12, HYPNOSIS AND THE REMISSION OF CANCER

Barber, T. *Hypnosis: A Scientific Approach*. New York: Van Nostrand Reinhold, 1969.

Barber, T., N. Spanos, and J. Chaves. *Hypnosis, Imagination and Human Potentialities*. New York: Pergamon, 1974.

Butler, B. The Use of Hypnosis in the Care of the Cancer Patient. *Cancer* 7 (1954): 1–14.

Cheek, D., and L. LeCron. *Clinical Hypnotherapy*. New York: Grune and Straton, 1968.

Clawson, T. A. The Hypnotic Control of Blood Flow and Pain: The Cure for Warts and the Potential for the Use of Hypnosis in the Treatment of Cancer. *American Journal of Clinical Hypnosis* 17 (1975): 160–69.

Evans, E. *A Psychological Study of Cancer*. New York: Dodd, Mead, 1926.

French, A. P. Treatment of Warts by Hypnosis. *American Journal of Obstetrics and Gynecology* 116 (1973): 887–88.

Erickson, M. Naturalistic Techniques of Hypnosis. *American Journal of Clinical Hypnosis* 1 (1958): 3–8.

Gill, M., and M. Brenman. *Hypnosis and Related States*. New York: International Universities Press, 1959.

Haley, J. *Uncommon Therapy*. New York: Norton, 1973.

Hall, H. R. Hypnosis and the Immune System: A Review with Implications for Cancer and the Psychology of Healing. *Journal of Clinical Hypnosis* 25 (1982-1983): 2-3.

Hilgard, J. *Personality and Hypnosis*. Chicago: University of Chicago Press, 1970.

Lansky, P. S. The Possibility of Hypnosis as an Aid in Cancer Therapy. *Perspectives in Biology and Medicine* 25 (1982): 496-501.

Meares, A. A. Working Hypothesis as to the Nature of Hypnosis. American Medical Association In Chicago: *Archives of Neurology and Psychiatry*. 77 (1957): 549-55.

Paul, G. L. Physiological Effects of Relaxation Training and Hypnotic Suggestion. *Journal of Abnormal Psychology* 74 (1969): 425-37.

Reich, W. Activist and Traditional Approaches in Psychiatry. *American Journal of Psychiatry* 130 (1973): 825-26.

Sheehan, P. W. Hypnosis and Processes of Imagination. In *Hypnosis: Developments in Research and New Perspectives*. New York: Wiley, 1983.

CHAPTER 13, METABOLIC THERAPIES AND THE REMISSION OF CANCER

Bradford, R. W., with M. Culbert. *Now That You Have Cancer*. Los Altos, CA: Choice Publications, 1977.

Bricklin, M. *Natural Healing*. Emmaus, PA: Rodale Press, 1976.

Brody, J., with A. Holleb. *You Can Fight Cancer and Win*. New York: McGraw-Hill, 1977.

Culbert, M. *Freedom from Cancer*. New York: Pocket Books, 1976.

Deverell, D. *How I Healed My Cancer Holistically*. Manhattan Beach, CA: Mother Earth News, 1978.

Dubos, R. Bolstering the Body Against Disease. *Journal of the Nutritional Academy*. 2 (1976):54.

Fahey, J. C. Cancer and the Immune Response. *Journal of the Nutritional Academy*. 2 (1981): 38.

Gerson, M. *A Cancer Therapy*. Del Mar, CA: Totality Books, 1958.

Glasser, R. *The Body Is Hero*. New York: Random House, 1976.

Haught, S. J. *Has Dr. Max Gerson A True Cancer Cure?* North Hollywood, CA: London Press, 1962.

Holzer, H. *Beyond Medicine*. New York: Ballantine, 1973.

Israel, L. *Conquering Cancer*. New York: Random House, 1980.

Jaffe, D. *Healing from Within*. New York: Alfred A. Knopf, 1980.

Kelley, W. *One Answer to Cancer*. Beverly Hills, CA: International Association of Cancer Victims and Friends, 1974.

Krebs, Ernst, Jr., et al. "The Nature of Cancer." *Cancer Control Journal*, 2, No. 6, 1979: 45.

LeShan, L. L. *You Can Fight for Your Life*. New York: M. Evans and Company, 1976.

Livingston, V. *Cancer: A New Breakthrough*. San Diego, CA: Production House Publishers, 1972.

Passwater, R. *Cancer and its Nutritional Therapies*. New Canaan, CT: Keats Publishing Inc., 1978.

Rapaport, S. A. *Strike Back at Cancer: What to Do and Where to Go for the Best Medical Care*. Englewood Cliffs, NJ: Prentice-Hall, 1978.

Stauth, C. *Alternative Cancer Therapies*. Brookline Village, MA: New Age, 1978.

Tropp, J. *Cancer: A Healing Crisis*. Smithtown, NY: Exposition Press, 1980.

CHAPTER 15, ANOTHER WINNER

Deverell, D. *How I Cured Myself of Cancer Holistically*. Manhattan Beach, CA: Mother Earth News, 1978.

———. A Personal Cancer Cure. *Mother Earth News* (March–April 1979): 70–71.

Index

253

For physician referrals contact:

Albert Marchetti, M.D.
PO Box 214
Midtown Station
New York, NY 10018